P H Y S I C I A N S ' P R E S S

METABOLIC SYNDROME ESSENTIALS

David S. H. Bell, MD, FACE

Clinical Professor of Medicine
University of Alabama at Birmingham
Southside Endocrinology
Birmingham, AL

James H. O'Keefe, MD, FACC

Director of Preventive Cardiology
Mid-America Heart Institute
Professor of Medicine
University of Missouri
Kansas City, MO

2011

W9-CDS-315

JONES & BARTLETT
L E A R N I N G

World Headquarters
Jones & Bartlett Learning
40 Tall Pine Drive
Sudbury, MA 01776
978-443-5000
info@jblearning.com
www.jblearning.com

Jones & Bartlett Learning
Canada
6339 Ormindale Way
Mississauga, Ontario L5V 1J2
Canada

Jones & Bartlett Learning
International
Barb House, Barb Mews
London W6 7PA
United Kingdom

Jones & Bartlett Learning books and products are available through most bookstores and online booksellers. To contact Jones & Bartlett Learning directly, call 800-832-0034, fax 978-443-8000, or visit our website, www.jblearning.com.

Substantial discounts on bulk quantities of Jones & Bartlett Learning publications are available to corporations, professional associations, and other qualified organizations. For details and specific discount information, contact the special sales department at Jones & Bartlett Learning via the above contact information or send an email to specialsales@jblearning.com.

The authors, editor, and publisher have made every effort to provide accurate information. However, they are not responsible for errors, omissions, or for any outcomes related to the use of the contents of this book and take no responsibility for the use of the products and procedures described. Treatments and side effects described in this book may not be applicable to all people; likewise, some people may require a dose or experience a side effect that is not described herein. Drugs and medical devices are discussed that may have limited availability controlled by the Food and Drug Administration (FDA) for use only in a research study or clinical trial. Research, clinical practice, and government regulations often change the accepted standard in this field. When consideration is being given to use of any drug in the clinical setting, the healthcare provider or reader is responsible for determining FDA status of the drug, reading the package insert, and reviewing prescribing information for the most up-to-date recommendations on dose, precautions, and contraindications, and determining the appropriate usage for the product. This is especially important in the case of drugs that are new or seldom used.

Production Credits
Executive Publisher: Christopher Davis
Senior Acquisitions Editor: Alison Hankey
Editorial Assistant: Sara Cameron
Associate Marketing Manager: Katie Hennessy
Production Director: Amy Rose
Associate Production Editor: Jessica deMartin
V.P., Manufacturing and Inventory Control: Therese Connell
Composition: diacriTech, Chennai, India
Cover Design: Scott Moden
Cover Image Credit: © Sebastian Kaulitzki/ShutterStock, Inc.
Printing and Binding: Cenveo
Cover Printing: Cenveo

ISBN-13: 978-0-7637-8178-1

6048

Printed in the United States of America
14 13 12 11 10   10 9 8 7 6 5 4 3 2 1

David S. H. Bell, MD, FACE, is a native of Northern Ireland where he graduated from Queens University Medical School. After immigrating to Canada and completing training in endocrinology, 2 years in private practice, and 2 years on faculty at Temple University Medical School, Dr. Bell joined the faculty at the University of Alabama Medical School where he was a professor of medicine for 25 years before retirement to private practice in 2005.

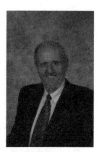

Dr. Bell has published over 290 articles in referenced medical journals and 3 books including *Diet For Life*, the story of his own weight loss. He is also a reviewer for many general medicine and endocrine journals, has served on multiple editorial boards, and has delivered invited lectures in Italy, Ireland, Canada, Australia, New Zealand, India, Singapore, Korea, Taiwan, Malaysia, the Philippines, and Puerto Rico. He has been active in many clinical interventional trials for the treatment of diabetes and its complications. In addition, his clinical abilities have been recognized by his peers with his inclusion in the "Best Doctors in America" and "America's Top Doctors" since 2001, "Best Doctors for Men" in *Men's Health* in 2007, and "Best Doctors for Women" in *Women's Health* in 2008. In 2001, he was presented the Distinguished Clinician Award by the American College of Endocrinology for outstanding contributions as a master educator and clinician, and in 2002, the Seale Harris Award by the Southern Medical Association for superior contributions to the art and science of diabetes and endocrinology.

James H. O'Keefe, MD, FACC, is director of preventive cardiology at the Mid America Heart Institute and professor of medicine at the University of Missouri in Kansas City. His postgraduate training included a cardiology fellowship at the Mayo Clinic in Rochester, Minnesota. Dr. O'Keefe has contributed more than 180 articles to medical literature and has authored numerous books on cardiovascular medicine, including *Dyslipidemia Essentials, Diabetes Essentials,* and *The Complete Guide to ECGs*. He lectures extensively on the role of therapeutic lifestyle changes and drug therapy in cardiovascular risk reduction and has authored the best-selling consumer health book, *The Forever Young Diet and Lifestyle*. He is actively involved in patient care, research, and teaching.

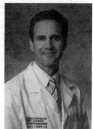

TABLE OF CONTENTS

Table of Contents

ABBREVIATIONS

5-AMPK	5-AMP-activated protein kinase	LDL	low-density lipoprotein
ACS	acute coronary syndrome	LH	luteinizing hormone
ADMA	asymmetric dimethyl arginine	LHRH	luteinizing hormone releasing hormone
AD	Alzheimer's disease		
ApoB	apolipoprotein B	LVH	left ventricular hypertrophy
ATP	adenosine triphosphate	MI	myocardial infarction
BMI	body mass index	MetSyn	metabolic syndrome
BPH	benign prostatic hypertrophy	NAFLD	nonalcoholic fatty liver disease
CKD	chronic kidney disease	NASH	nonalcoholic steatohepatitis
CV	cardiovascular	PAD	peripheral vascular disease
CPT-1	carnitine palmotransferase-1	PAI_1	plasminogen activator inhibitor
CRP	C-reactive protein	PCOS	polycystic ovary syndrome
DPP-4	dipeptyl peptidase-4	PGC-1	peroxisome-proliferator-activated receptor gamma coactivator
DES	drug-eluting stent		
ESRD	end-stage renal disease		
FFA	free fatty acid	PPAR	peroxisome-proliferator-activated receptor
FSH	follicular stimulating hormone		
GLP_1	glucagon-like peptide	RAAS	renin-angiotensin-aldosterone system
GRH	gonadotrophin releasing hormone		
		SAS	sleep apnea syndrome
HCV	hepatitis C virus	TNF-α	tumor necrosis factor-alpha
HDL	high-density lipoprotein	TPA	tissue plasminogen activator
HF	heart failure	TZD	thiazolidinedione
HH	hypogonadotrophic hypogonadism	VEGF	vascular endothelial growth factor
IGF_1	insulin-like growth factor 1	VLDL	very low density lipoprotein
IL-6	interleukin 6	VSMC	vascular smooth muscle cell

Chapter 1

Introduction to Metabolic Syndrome

DEFINITION

Metabolic syndrome (MetSyn) is an inflammatory, hypercoagulable state associated with excess peritoneal and hepatic fat, oxidative stress, endothelial dysfunction, hypertension, a characteristic dyslipidemia [low HDL (high-density lipoprotein) levels, high triglyceride levels, and small dense LDL (low-density lipoprotein) and HDL particles], and hyperinsulinemia. Because of these features, MetSyn is associated with an increased prevalence of type 2 diabetes, cardiovascular (CV) risk factors, atherosclerosis, and CV events.

HISTORY OF METABOLIC SYNDROME

The concept that tissue resistance to insulin plays a role in diabetes and other disease states is not new. In fact, this hypothesis has been proposed multiple times since it was first put forward approximately 70 years ago. However, it was not until the development of an insulin immunoassay by Bearson and Yallow almost 50 years ago that the hypothesis could be proven.

Reaven extended the concept of insulin resistance and its relationship to diabetes and CV risk and named it syndrome X, which he defined as hypertriglyceridemia, low HDL levels, and hypertension. He hypothesized that this constellation of risks plays an important role in non–insulin-dependent diabetes and coronary artery disease (CAD). Over the next 6 years he added to the syndrome the presence of smaller, denser LDL particles and abnormalities of fibrinolysis.

At times, MetSyn has been referred to as Reaven's syndrome and insulin-resistance syndrome, but it is now most commonly referred to as MetSyn. The clinical criteria for diagnosing MetSyn were definitively established by the Third Report of the National Cholesterol Education Program/Adult Treatment Panel III (NCEP/ATP III). However, the International Diabetes Federation (IDF) later amended the clinical criteria so that central obesity, as defined by an increased waist circumference, must be present for a diagnosis of MetSyn.

DIAGNOSIS OF INSULIN-RESISTANCE SYNDROME

Although a high fasting serum insulin level is diagnostic of MetSyn, the test is unnecessary and associated with many false-negative results. The reason for the unreliability of this test is that insulin assays are not well standardized and the liver periodically withdraws insulin from the blood, resulting in transiently lower serum insulin levels, thereby inappropriately ruling out the diagnosis of MetSyn. C-peptide, the remnant protein that remains when insulin is formed from its precursor proinsulin, has a much longer half-life than insulin. Thus, measurement of serum C-peptide is a better diagnostic test. In most cases, measurement of C-peptide is unnecessary, because the diagnosis of insulin resistance can and should be made clinically.

As per the NCEP/ATP III criteria, a clinical diagnosis of the MetSyn can be made if any three of the following five risk factors are present:

1. A waist circumference measured at the level of the iliac crests that is greater than 35 inches (89 cm) in a woman or 40 inches (102 cm) in a man

2. An HDL cholesterol less than 50 mg/dL in a woman or less than 40 mg/dL in a man

3. A fasting triglyceride level greater than 150 mg/dL

4. Diagnosed hypertension or a blood pressure above 130/80 mm Hg

5. A fasting serum glucose greater than 100 mg/dL or previously diagnosed type 2 diabetes

Based on these criteria, almost 24% of the American adult population and 44% of those older than age 60 have MetSyn. This means that there are at least 47 million people in the United States with MetSyn, of whom only 40% will ever develop diabetes. However, the remaining 60%, despite remaining nondiabetic, will still have a two- to fivefold increase in cardiac events.

PROBLEMS IN DIAGNOSING METABOLIC SYNDROME

Although a clinical diagnosis is the gold standard for diagnosing MetSyn, a high suspicion for the presence of MetSyn can be obtained from a fasting lipid profile. The fasting triglyceride-to-HDL ratio correlates well with the gold standard for diagnosing MetSyn–the Insulin Clamp Study. If this ratio exceeds 3.5, then it is highly likely that MetSyn (and insulin resistance) is present.

Unfortunately, MetSyn is underdiagnosed, because in most clinical situations waist circumference is either not measured or is measured incorrectly (the belt size will often markedly underestimate the true waist circumference, particularly in males). This excludes what is generally considered the most important diagnostic criterion for the diagnosis of MetSyn. In these situations, utilization of the triglyceride-to-HDL ratio is helpful.

Another problem with waist circumference is that, particularly in people of Asian ethnicity, MetSyn is often present in a thin individual with a "normal" waist circumference. Because the waist circumference is greater in a tall person than it is in a small person, it is important that waist circumference be adjusted for height. Ideally, the waist circumference should be half the height, and a waist-to-height ratio greater than 0.55 is abnormal. Different criteria for the waist circumference in Asian persons have been established by the International Diabetes Federation to facilitate the diagnosis of MetSyn in these generally thin persons.

OTHER CLUES TO THE PRESENCE OF METABOLIC SYNDROME

The presence of acanthosis nigricans is a "giveaway" as a marker of MetSyn. Often described as "the ring around the collar that will not wash off," acanthosis nigricans is seldom seen in persons of European origin, but it is common in Native Americans, Asian Americans, African Americans, and Hispanic Americans (in the latter, the prevalence of acanthosis nigricans is as high as 12% by age 13). Acanthosis nigricans is dark in color and velvety to the touch. It is most easily seen on the neck but it may also present in the axillary and inguinal regions.

Further clinical clues for the presence of MetSyn are the presence of polycystic ovary syndrome (PCOS), nonalcoholic hepatic steatosis or steatohepatitis, albuminuria, and an elevated uric acid level or a history of gout.

Chapter 2
Etiology of Metabolic Syndrome

GENETIC FACTORS AND MITOCHONDRIAL FUNCTION

Genetic factors account for at least 50% of the etiology of MetSyn. The genetic defect is now thought to reside in the mitochondria, where oxidative phosphorylation is reduced by 30% due to decreased expression of peroxisome proliferator-activated receptor (PPAR) gamma coactivator (PGC-1), a coactivator of the PPAR gamma receptor. As a result of the decreased expression of PGC-1, the mitochondria are not only anatomically smaller but are physiologically less efficient. Decreased mitochondrial function allows triglycerides to accumulate in the cytoplasm and build up in tissues such as voluntary muscle, the liver, and the myocardium. Triglyceride accumulation in pancreatic beta cells is also a feature of MetSyn. Because mitochondrial defects are inherited exclusively from the mother, this would explain why type 2 diabetes is much more commonly present on the maternal rather than on the paternal side of the family in diabetic patients.

Voluntary muscle in normoglycemic subjects without insulin resistance has a high mitochondrial content, resulting in a high capacity for lipid oxidation and low myocellular lipid levels. The metabolism of triglycerides depends on the ability of carnitine palmotransferase-1 (CPT-1) to transport triglycerides into the mitochondria. In the insulin-resistant subject, the activity of CPT-1 is decreased, causing triglycerides to accumulate in the cytoplasm. The accumulation of triglycerides in the cytoplasm of the cardiomyocyte, hepatocyte, and pancreatic beta cells leads to cardiomyopathy, fatty liver disease, and diabetes, respectively.

The genetic predisposition to insulin resistance in the voluntary muscle and liver—the cardinal features of MetSyn—is worsened by the loss of the muscle mass that occurs with aging, abdominal obesity, lack of aerobic exercise, infection, anxiety, depression, smoking, sleep deprivation, corticosteroids, and hypogonadism.

However, even in the presence of severe insulin resistance only 40% of subjects go on to develop type 2 diabetes, because until substantially decreased insulin secretion becomes manifest the individual generally does not become overtly diabetic. In fact, of the 10 genes associated with type 2 diabetes that have, to date, been identified, 8 are associated with defective insulin secretion and only 2 are associated with insulin resistance. However, those insulin-resistant MetSyn subjects who do not develop diabetes still have an excessive risk of CV disease and CV events.

THE ROLE OF PERITONEAL FAT

MetSyn is associated with the male pattern of fat distribution, where the fat is abdominal rather than on the buttocks and thighs, which are relatively thin (apple shape). The fat distribution of the obese female, where fat is deposited in the buttocks and thighs (pear shape), is not associated with MetSyn. Buttock and thigh fat are subcutaneous and are primarily storage fat with a low metabolic activity, thus they are not associated with MetSyn (Figure 2.1).

Interestingly, bigger thighs are associated with a lower risk of heart disease or premature death. In one study, both men and women whose thigh circumference was less than 55 cm (22 inches) had a two-fold increased risk for a cardiac event or death. The underlying explanation for this finding likely relates to the disturbed hormonal milieu (higher cortisol and catecholamine levels, with suboptimal sex hormones) found in individuals with MetSyn, which predisposes one to more fat deposition in the liver and peritoneal cavity and less in the thighs.

To be associated with MetSyn, abdominal fat must be deposited in excess in the peritoneal cavity, where the adipocytes situated in omental, mesenteric, retroperitoneal, and perinephric fat are more metabolically active (Figure 2.2). However, not every obese patient has increased peritoneal fat and MetSyn, and not every thin patient escapes excessive

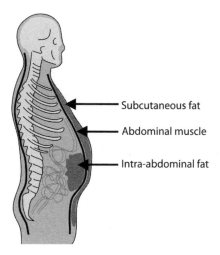

- Subcutaneous fat
- Abdominal muscle
- Intra-abdominal fat

Figure 2.1. Abdominal Adiposity: The Critical Adipose Depot

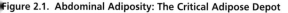

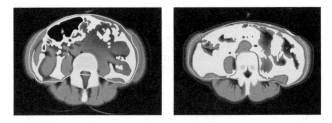

Figure 2.2. Visceral Fat Distribution: Normal vs. Type 2 Diabetes

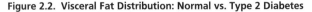

Courtesy of Wilfred Y. Fujimoto, MD.

peritoneal fat and MetSyn. As a result, 40% of those persons with a body mass index (BMI) greater than 35 do not have MetSyn, whereas 6% of those with a BMI below 25 meet criteria for MetSyn.

An example of the obese subject without MetSyn is the Japanese Sumo wrestler who has a normal visceral-to-subcutaneous fat ratio because he partakes in an intensive and lengthy daily exercise program. In contrast, recent studies of professional American football players have shown that MetSyn is present in approximately 22% of lineman, virtually all of whom are obese despite a regimen that includes hours of daily exercise.

An example of the thin subject with MetSyn is the Asian individual with type 2 diabetes. MetSyn is very prevalent on the Indian subcontinent and is particularly prevalent in patients who have moved from a rural to an urban environment and have adopted an urbanized life- style. These lifestyle changes cause an increase in peritoneal fat, causing their BMI to rise above 23 and their waist to expand to greater than 34 inches (86 cm). MetSyn manifests itself early in these relatively "thin" persons because of a genetic predisposition to insulin resistance.

Not all subcutaneous fat is metabolically inactive. Abdominal subcutaneous fat is divided by a facial plane into outer and inner layers. The inner layer of abdominal sub- cutaneous fat is much more metabolically active and functions in much the same way as peritoneal fat. The probable reason for this is that, like peritoneal adipocytes, these deeper subcutaneous adipocytes are infiltrated by macrophages and have direct access to the portal circulation.

Increased free fatty acids (FFAs) are released into the portal circulation from the increased numbers of metabolically active peritoneal adipocytes. Increased FFA levels lead to hepatic resistance to the action of insulin, increased hepatic glucose and triglyceride pro- duction, lower hepatic HDL production, and increased storage of FFAs as triglycerides in the cytoplasm of the hepatocytes. Excessive FFAs entering and later exiting the portal circulation and entering the systemic circulation adds to the increased cytoplasmic triglyceride levels of the myocytes, cardiomyocytes, and pancreatic beta cells, leading to insulin resistance, cardio- myopathy, and pancreatic beta cell dysfunction.

Peritoneal fat accounts for 20% of total body fat mass in males and 6% in females. Higher testosterone levels in females increases the percentage of peritoneal fat, as does testosterone replacement therapy in hypogonadal males. The increased volume of peritoneal fat that occurs with increased testosterone levels is caused by increases in the number of androgen receptors present in the nucleus of the peritoneal adipocyte when compared with subcutaneous adiptocytes.

In the autosomal-dominant Dunnigan-Kobberling syndrome, a person experiences the total loss of subcutaneous fat in the limbs, trunk, and breasts, retaining subcutaneous fat only in the face and neck. In this syndrome, compensatory deposition of fat in the peritoneal cavity and the liver results in severe insulin resistance. Similarly, lipodystrophy syndromes associated with HIV infection and/or antiretroviral therapy are associated with the redistribution of fat into the peritoneal cavity and liver, severe insulin resistance, and an increased prevalence of type 2 diabetes.

The increased metabolic activity of peritoneal fat when compared with subcutaneous fat is due to the presence of a higher density of beta-adrenergic receptors and a lower density of alpha-1 adrenergic receptors on the surface of the peritoneal adipocyte, which leads to increased catecholamine-induced lipolysis and an increased release of FFAs into the portal circulation. The increased inflammatory activity associated with the peritoneal fat is due to infiltration of peritoneal and hepatic fat with macrophages.

ADIPOCYTOKINES

Macrophages are recruited from the bone marrow in proportion to the number of peritoneal adipocytes so that the greater the number of peritoneal adipocytes the greater the recruitment of macrophages to the peritoneal fat. These adipocytes produce excess inflammatory adipocytokines due to infiltration of macrophages in a corona surrounding the peritoneal and hepatic adipocytes and crosstalk between macrophages and adipocytes. As a result of this excessive production of adipocytokines by the peritoneal adipocytes, Met-Syn is associated with a chronic low-grade inflammation. The crosstalk that leads to inflammation within the adipocyte also results in increased resistance to the action of insulin on the adipocyte, increased lipolysis, and the release of FFAs into the portal circulation. The inflammation within the peritoneal fat results in increased release of inflammatory cytokines.

In animal studies, the adipocytokine resistin (the role of which is controversial in humans) is produced in excess by peritoneal fat, and this excess production occurs whether the etiology of the obesity is genetic or induced by excessive calorie intake in a genetically thin animal. Administration of exogenous recombinant resistin to an insulin-sensitive animal impairs the action of insulin on muscle and raises glucose levels. In contrast, administration of antibodies to resistin improves insulin sensitivity and lowers glucose levels in insulin-resistant animals (Figure 2.3).

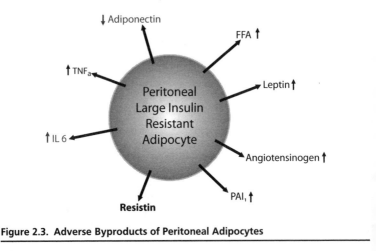

Figure 2.3. Adverse Byproducts of Peritoneal Adipocytes

TUMOR NECROSIS FACTOR-ALPHA (TNF-α)

Although the role of resistin in humans is questionable, the role of tumor necrosis factor-alpha (TNF-α) in humans is well established. TNF-α produced by peritoneal adipocytes increases the release of FFAs, leading to higher portal FFA levels. On reaching the systemic circulation, elevated FFA levels not only decrease insulin sensitivity but also increase coagulability and the risk of cardiac arrhythmias.

INTERLEUKIN-6 AND C-REACTIVE PROTEIN

Interleukin-6 (IL-6) is also produced in excess by the increased mass of macrophage-infiltrated peritoneal adipocytes. Although IL-6 is produced by multiple tissues, at least a third of total IL-6 production is from adipocytes, particularly peritoneal adipocytes. Increased production and release of IL-6 from peritoneal adipocytes on entering the portal circulation leads to an increase hepatic production of C-reactive protein (CRP).

CRP was first identified as a cytokine produced in excess during an acute-phase reaction induced by a bacterial infection. CRP is protective against bacterial infections, such as *Pneumococcus* infections, by being able to perforate the bacterial wall. Although a marked elevation of CRP in a bacterial infection is protective and beneficial, a chronic low-grade elevation of CRP is associated with increased CV disease. Chronic elevation of CRP is considered a marker of both low-grade systemic inflammation and inflammation within the atheromatous plaque, which increases the likelihood that the plaque will rupture and cause a cardiac event. Indeed, any distant inflammation (joints, intestine, etc.) may stimulate inflammation within an atheromatous plaque. CRP, in addition to being a marker of inflammatory atherosclerosis, may also play an active role in the formation of atheromatous plaques. At autopsy, when coronary arteries are stained for CRP, it is present in the atheromatous plaques, including the smallest and earliest plaques; it is not found in the healthy plaque-free endothelium of the coronary arteries.

Monocytes, owing to a surface receptor for CRP, are drawn toward and more easily penetrate the endothelium of the arterial wall when CRP is present. Therefore, CRP is not just a marker of chronic low-grade inflammation and inflammation within an atheromatous plaque; it may also play a very active role in the formation of as well as the rupture of an atheromatous plaque. Treating MetSyn with a thiazolidinedione (TZD) has been shown to significantly lower CRP levels even when concurrent statin therapy is being utilized. Because at least one TZD has been shown to decelerate the increase in the volume of both coronary and carotid artery atheroma and to decrease cardiac events, lowering of CRP and inflammation with a TZD in MetSyn subjects plays at least a partial role in the positive CV effects of these drugs.

In addition to its effects that are mediated through hepatic CRP production, IL-6 has other direct deleterious effects on the CV system. IL-6 is prothrombotic, stimulating the production of fibrinogen by the liver and increasing the expression of tissue factors in both monocytes and endothelial cells, which leads to activation of the coagulation cascade. Through its effect on the endothelium, IL-6 also adversely affects endothelial function, which results in vasoconstriction, thrombosis, and deposition of atheroma. Therefore, both directly and indirectly, excessive IL-6 results in inflammation, endothelial dysfunction, and atherogenesis.

PLASMINOGEN ACTIVATOR INHIBITOR AND ANGIOTENSINOGEN

Plasminogen activator inhibitor (PAI_1) is produced in excess by peritoneal adipocytes. It works directly against tissue plasminogen activator (TPA) and decreases the formation of plasmin from plasminogen. Decreased plasmin in the systemic circulation slows the breakdown of fibrin, decreasing the lysis of clots and therefore increasing the frequency and severity of thromboembolic events. In addition, plasmin is needed in the vessel wall to break down and remove collagen from atheromatous plaques in order to make room for vascular smooth muscle cells to enter the plaque and replace the collagen tissue. Entry of these vascular smooth muscle cells into the atheromatous plaque results in plaque stabilization so that plaque rupture and CV events are less likely to occur. Elevated levels of PAI_1 within the vessel wall have been documented in both MetSyn and type 2 diabetes. TZDs have been shown to reduce PAI_1 levels in patients with MetSyn, which could at least partially explain the decreases in CV events that have been documented with the TZD pioglitazone (see Chapter 4).

Peritoneal adipocytes also produce angiotensinogen, which is the substrate acted upon by renin to form angiotensin I and subsequently angiotensin II. The excess production of angiotensinogen may have a role in the increased frequency of hypertension that occurs in MetSyn (see Chapter 3). Angiotensin II levels have been shown to be increased in MetSyn, and increased angiotensin II levels are associated with increases in inflammation, oxidative stress, endothelial dysfunction, formation of atheroma, and cardiac events.

11β-HYDROXYSTEROID DEHYDROGENASE AND LEPTIN

11β-hydroxysteroid dehydrogenase (11β-OHSD-1) is an enzyme that facilitates the conversion of metabolically inactive cortisone to metabolically active cortisol. It is produced in excess by peritoneal adipocytes. Therefore, excess production of 11β-OHSD-1 could account for the "Cushingoid appearance" that occurs in many subjects with MetSyn. However, the activity of 11β-OHSD-1 is more active at a local level than it is systemically, thus testing for Cushing's syndrome in these patients is almost invariably negative. Transgenic mice given the gene for 11β-OHSD-1 develop hyperphagia, weight gain, insulin resistance, and diabetes, probably due to increased local cortisol production.

Although excess leptin production is more a feature of excess production by subcutaneous rather excess peritoneal adipocytes, leptin levels are also increased in MetSyn. Increased leptin levels are associated in most, but not all, studies with increased insulin resistance, worsened endothelial function, and hypertension due to increased activity of the sympathetic nervous system. Lowering of leptin levels is associated with an improvement in the features of MetSyn. In addition to its ability to increase appetite and hyperphagia, leptin has also been shown to increase the activity of the alpha cells of the pancreatic islets, resulting in increased glucagon release. Increased glucagon release in combination with insulin resistance increases the risk of developing type 2 diabetes and worsens glycemic control in those patients with established diabetes. Leptin has also been associated with hematopoiesis, vascular endothelial proliferation, and angiogenesis. Immunologically, leptin also causes proliferation of T lymphocytes.

ADIPONECTIN

At present, the only adipocytokine produced by peritoneal and hepatic adipocytes that is known to be beneficial to humans is adiponectin. Lower serum levels of adiponectin are associated with obesity, MetSyn, type 2 diabetes, and CAD. Decreasing levels of adiponectin precede the development of MetSyn, and adiponectin levels climb rapidly when MetSyn is treated. Adiponectin is believed to improve the features of MetSyn by accelerating the metabolism of FFAs and decreasing oxidative stress. In humans, the presence of MetSyn is characterized by insulin resistance, inflammation, increased oxidative stress, and endothelial dysfunction; all of these features are at least, in part, dependent on and positively associated with the ratio of IL-6 to adiponectin. As IL-6 levels increase and adiponectin levels decrease, insulin sensitivity deteriorates. Conversely, as IL-6 levels decrease and adiponectin levels increase, insulin sensitivity improves.

Adiponectin levels are higher in women, those with type 1 diabetes, thinner patients, and patients utilizing insulin sensitizers. Adiponectin levels are lower in men with type 2 diabetes, the obese, and those with lipodystrophy. The improvement in insulin sensitivity seen with increasing adiponectin levels has been shown to be associated with activation of the enzyme glycogen synthase. Activation of glycogen synthase increases cellular glucose uptake and FFA oxidation and decreases cytoplasmic triglyceride levels and hepatic glucose production.

Adiponectin has antiatherogenic effects that are mediated through reductions in each of the following steps in the atherosclerotic process: adhesion molecule levels, adhesion of monocytes to the endothelium, proliferation and migration of vascular smooth muscle cells into the endothelium, cytokine production by infiltrating monocytes, uptake of oxidized LDL by the macrophages, and foam cell formation.

However, adiponectin levels are often elevated with acute CV events, congestive heart failure (HF), and renal failure. This phenomenon has been called the "adiponectin paradox"; it probably represents the increased release of adiponectin due to tissue damage and the more advanced and severe stages of the underlying disease processes.

Metabolically, adiponectin also decreases the secretion of the tissue inhibitors of metalloproteinases, which results in decreases in both adipocyte hypertrophy and the number of peritoneal adipocytes.

CONCLUSION

Through genetic and environmental factors, excess peritoneal fat infiltrated with macrophages produces excessive FFAs and harmful adipocytokines and decreases production of the protective adipocytokine adiponectin. The net effect of this imbalance in adipocytokines is inflammation, oxidative stress, endothelial dysfunction, insulin insensitivity, excess coagulation, atherosclerosis, type 2 diabetes, and adverse CV events.

Chapter 3

Cardiac Risk Factors Associated with Metabolic Syndrome

HYPERTENSION

Hypertension is one of the diagnostic features of MetSyn. Seventy-five percent of those with type 2 diabetes are hypertensive, and 50% of subjects with hypertension have the MetSyn. Furthermore, MetSyn subjects with hypertension are "nondippers"; that is, they do not experience the normal physiological drop in blood pressure during sleeping hours that is caused by persistently and pathologically elevated catecholamine levels during sleep. Nondipping is also associated with an increased rate of CV events, particularly those occurring between midnight and 6:00 A.M. Furthermore, because hypertension and sleep apnea (both of which are strongly associated with MetSyn) are among the most prevalent causes of atrial fibrillation, the majority of patients with atrial fibrillation (the most common cardiac arrhythmia requiring hospitalization and office visits) also have MetSyn.

Hyperinsulinemia associated with MetSyn stimulates the sympathetic nervous system via the renin-angiotensin-aldosterone system (RAAS) directly through activation of angiotensin II type 1 (AT_1) receptors and indirectly by stimulation of the RAAS via increased catecholamine levels. Insulin causes the body to retain salt and water; thus hyperinsulinemia, through its action on the kidney's distal tubules, increases sodium retention and total body sodium. In addition to increased sodium content, the calcium content of the vascular smooth muscle cells (VSMCs) also increases with MetSyn. The net result of elevations in VSMC sodium and calcium levels is an increase in VSMC tone, peripheral arterial resistance, and hypertension. In addition, if diabetes develops, as it does in 40% of MetSyn subjects, hyperglycemia exacerbates sodium retention, because one molecule of sodium is also absorbed for every molecule of glucose filtered and reabsorbed by the renal tubule. Furthermore, the increase in peritoneal fat mass, which is invariably associated with MetSyn, is associated with increased production of angiotensinogen, the substrate for renin activity. Although lowering serum glucose will itself lower systolic blood pressure, concurrently lowering levels of insulin through therapeutic treatment of MetSyn will result in additional lowering.

Another factor in the etiology of hypertension associated with MetSyn is increased FFA levels. In a study designed to simulate MetSyn, obese normotensive type 2 diabetic patients had their FFA levels increased by the administration of intravenous intralipid with heparin over 48 hours. Subjects with increased FFA levels experienced increases in their systolic blood pressure by 5 mm Hg compared with normotensive type 2 diabetic subjects who received a similar volume of intravenous fluid in the form of saline with heparin. In addition, flow-mediated dilatation (a measure of endothelial function) decreased by 18% and high-sensitivity CRP (hs-CRP, a measure of inflammation) increased by 110% after the intralipid infusion. No changes in renin activity or aldosterone levels were observed in this study.

Although hypertension alone often leads to left ventricular hypertrophy (LVH), MetSyn potentiates this trophic effect on the myocardium, in part due to high levels of insulin, which is a growth factor. The Hypertension Generic Epidemiology (Hyper GEN) study found that MetSyn was associated with increased ventricular mass and wall thickness. The development of type 2 diabetes caused a further increase in LVH. However, even at the time of diagnosis of diabetes, LVH, as assessed by echocardiography, was present in 32% of nonhypertensive subjects due to preexisting MetSyn; in unselected type 2 diabetic subjects, 71% had LVH. It should be noted, at least in African American subjects, that the presence of LVH is associated with a mortality higher than that which occurs with multiple-vessel CAD or left ventricular systolic dysfunction.

DYSLIPIDEMIA

The lipid pattern of MetSyn is characterized by high triglycerides and a low HDL cholesterol level. Additional features are an increased number of LDL particles accompanied by an elevated apolipoprotein B (ApoB) cholesterol level (one ApoB per LDL particle) and normal or only slightly elevated total and calculated LDL cholesterol levels. The feature of MetSyn that has the greatest potential for atherogenesis and adverse CV events is the decreased size of both the LDL and HDL particles. In MetSyn, total and LDL cholesterol levels are no higher than levels seen in the population without MetSyn, because even though the number of LDL particles is increased the LDL particles are smaller and denser, which results in the total and LDL cholesterol levels being relatively normal.

The major cause of the small size of both the LDL and HDL particles that characterizes MetSyn is the presentation of triglyceride-rich very low-density lipoprotein (VLDL) particles to increased hepatic lipase activity, resulting in increased formation of both small dense LDL and HDL particles (Figure 3.1).

The increased number of smaller and denser LDL particles that occurs in MetSyn is associated with increased atherogenesis. This is because the small size of the LDL particle facilitates penetration of the arterial endothelium and entry into the subendothelial space where these small dense particles are more easily oxidized and, especially if glycosylated, more easily picked up by the scavenger receptor on the macrophage to initiate and facilitate atherogenesis (Figure 3.2).

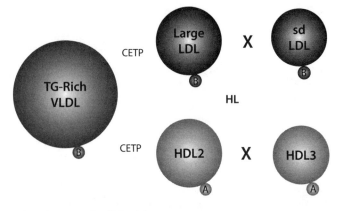

Figure 3.1. Large vs. Small Particles

CETP = cholesterol ester transferase protein; HL = hepatic lipase; LPL = lipoprotein lipase.

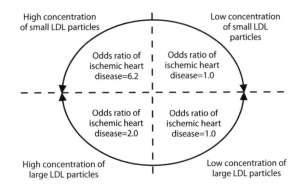

Figure 3.2. Small, Dense, LDL Particles as a Predictor of Ischemic Heart Disease

Source: Lamarche B, et al. Small, Dense Low-Density Lipoprotein Particles as a Predictor of the the Risk of Ischemic Heart Disease in Men: Prospective Results From the Quebec Cardiovascular Study. Clinical Investigation And Report. *Circulation.* 1997;95:69.

The small dense HDL particle, owing to its reduced capacity for reverse cholesterol transportation, is less cardioprotective than the larger HDL particle. In addition, the small dense HDL particle has less anti-inflammatory and anti-oxidant effects, which results in decreased improvement of endothelial function and less protection from oxidation of LDL particles. Furthermore, the smaller and denser HDL particles are more rapidly metabolized by the liver, which results in decreased longevity of these particles and, as a result, lower total HDL levels.

Therefore, in MetSyn the activity of hepatic lipase on triglyceride-rich VLDL particles is increased, resulting in the formation of small dense LDL and HDL particles. This causes the formation of larger numbers of atherogenic LDL particles and proportionally more small dense HDL particles that are shorter lived and less cardioprotective.

Improving MetSyn with a TZD results in increases in both HDL and LDL particle size without an increase in the number of particles. Because of the increased size of the LDL particles, the calculated LDL and total cholesterol levels increase, providing a false impression of worsening dyslipidemia. Therefore, the use of a TZD in no way interferes with, and indeed is complementary to, the action of a statin, which in most cases only lowers the total number of LDL particles without changing the particle size. Of the available statins, only atorvastatin and rosuvastatin have been shown to minimally increase LDL particle size, whereas all TZDs will substantially increase LDL particle size.

The effects of the available TZDs on the lipid profile differ. Although both rosiglitazone and pioglitazone increase total HDL levels as well as HDL and LDL particle sizes, pioglitazone is more effective in lowering triglyceride levels. However, the major difference between the two available TZDs is that pioglitazone decreases the number of LDL particles, whereas rosiglitazone increases the number of the LDL particles. This difference could explain the differences that these TZDs have on cardiac events (see Chapter 4). However, the differences in the lipid profile effects may not totally explain the differences in cardiac events that occur with these two TZDs (see Chapter 4). The expression of 26 genes is increased with both rosiglitazone and pioglitazone through activation of the PPAR-gamma receptor. Rosiglitazone exclusively increases the expression of an additional 5 genes, whereas pioglitazone uniquely increases the expression of 12 additional genes. Thus, differences in the lipid profile with the two available TZDs may simply be a marker for differences between these drugs on gene expression rather than a cause for the differences in cardiac events.

From a clinical perspective, the association of small dense LDL and HDL particles with cardiac events and longevity has been illustrated by three studies. The first, a cross-sectional study of Ashkenazi Jews, their offspring, and a control group (from the Framingham Study) showed that larger LDL and HDL particle sizes could explain the increased longevity of the Ashkenazi.

Similarly, it was noted that individuals with increased life expectancy in a small Italian town had a genetic proband that was associated with a low total HDL level and larger HDL particle size. In these subjects, the increase in HDL particle size is caused by a single genetic amino acid substitution that leads to dimerization and increased HDL particle size. This larger HDL particle (now called HDL Milano) was later shown in humans to decrease atheroma volume and improve clinical outcomes in patients following acute coronary syndrome (ACS) when administered intravenously weekly for 5 weeks.

That HDL particle size is associated with cardiac events was clearly shown in the HATS study, where the combined effects of administering simvastatin and niacin resulted not only in an angiographically assessed decrease in coronary artery atherosclerosis, but also unexpectedly decreased CV events. However, when the antioxidants beta carotene, vitamin E, selenium, and vitamin C were used in combination with simvastatin and nicotinic acid, the deceleration in the progression of atheroma and the decrease in cardiac events were both blunted. After multivariate analysis, the blunting of atheroma formation and frequency of cardiac events was clearly shown to be associated with decreases in the concentration of larger HDL particles.

Increasing the total HDL cholesterol concentration is more difficult than lowering the LDL cholesterol concentration, but the rewards are greater: for every 1% decrease in LDL cardiac events are also decreased by 1%, but for every 1% increase in HDL cardiac events are decreased by 2% to 3%. HDL levels are increased by 2% to 8% with statins, 10% to 20% with fibrates, and 20% to 40% with niacin. In MetSyn patients with type 2 diabetes, therapy with a TZD can result in as much as a 35% increase in total HDL, particularly if the baseline HDL is below 35 mg/dL. Furthermore, the increase in total HDL that occurs with TZDs is mainly from the larger, cardioprotective HDL particles. The ability of a TZD to increase the volume of the larger HDL particles is a property that is shared with a few other drugs, which include niacin, estrogen, omega-3 fatty acids, and phenytoin.

Although an elevated triglyceride level is a marker for MetSyn, it was not shown to be a risk factor for cardiac events in studies such as the United Kingdom Prospective Diabetes Study (UKPDS), because triglycerides were no longer a risk factor after the total HDL cholesterol concentration was factored into the statistical analysis. However, a meta-analysis that included more than 16,000 hypertriglyceridemic subjects showed that when large numbers of subjects with elevated triglyceride levels were studied epidemiologically elevated triglyceride levels became an independent cardiac risk factor. The likely reason for this association is that elevated triglyceride levels include highly atherogenic particles, such as intermediate-density lipoproteins (IDLs) and small dense VLDL particles. Increases in the numbers of these particles can be detected by simply calculating the non-HDL cholesterol level. Furthermore, postprandial triglyceride levels (which are commonly present in the setting of MetSyn) are much more strongly correlated with oxidative stress, inflammation, atherosclerosis, and adverse CV events than are fasting triglycerides.

In the presence of hypertriglyceridemia, the NCEP/ATP III recommends that the non-HDL cholesterol level, rather than the calculated LDL level, be used for risk assessment. To calculate the non-HDL cholesterol level, the HDL cholesterol level is subtracted from the total cholesterol level, and it can be based on either a fasting or nonfasting specimen. The goal for non-HDL cholesterol is 30 mg/dL above the goal for the calculated LDL cholesterol level. Although, in general, the non-HDL cholesterol level is a better prognosticator for cardiac events than is the calculated LDL cholesterol level, in diabetic and/or MetSyn patients the non-HDL cholesterol is particularly important. This is because the non-HDL cholesterol level represents the sum of all of the atherogenic particles (LDL, IDL, and small dense VLDL) and is approximately as predictive of a cardiac event as directly measured ApoB levels. When MetSyn is treated with a TZD or omega-3 fatty acids (fish oil), the non-HDL cholesterol, in contrast to the calculated LDL cholesterol, decreases; this drop in non-HDL cholesterol is magnified when either of these agents is used in combination with a statin.

Therefore, MetSyn is associated with a lower total HDL level, increases in the numbers of small dense LDL and HDL particles, elevated non-HDL cholesterol levels, and hypertriglyceridemia. Therapeutic treatment of MetSyn, including diet and exercise, will at least partially reverse these abnormalities, especially when these therapies are utilized in conjunction with a statin.

COAGULOPATHY

The role of increased serum PAI_1 in decreasing fibrinolysis and increasing fibrin levels and thromboembolic events in MetSyn was described in an earlier section of this chapter. In addition, by sensitizing platelets to prostacyclin (PGI_2) and enhancing endothelial generation of nitric oxide and PGI_2, the increased insulin levels present in MetSyn increase platelet aggregation. Furthermore, in MetSyn there is a loss of platelet sensitivity to nitric oxide and PGI_2 so that platelets aggregate and adhere to the endothelium. The risk of thromboembolism in MetSyn is further increased because the levels of clotting factors VII and XII are also increased. The addition of chronic hyperglycemia not only further increases PAI_1 levels but also leads to the glycation of fibrin, which alters both its structure and function so that when clotting occurs the clots that are generated are denser and more resistant to fibrinolysis.

Thus, due to denser fibrin, decreased fibrinolysis, increased platelet aggregation, oxidative stress, and endothelial dysfunction, MetSyn is associated with increases in thromboembolic events.

INFLAMMATION

MetSyn is an inflammatory state associated with increases in the white cell count, amyloid and serum levels of IL-6, TNF-α, and CRP. CRP levels are generally elevated in MetSyn patients, and thus it is not mandatory to measure CRP in this setting. Furthermore, therapies that reduce inflammation and CRP levels [TZDs, metformin, statins, angiotensin II receptor blockers (ARBs), angiotensin-converting enzyme (ACE) inhibitors, aspirin, beta blockers] are often already being utilized in these patients. The inflammatory state associated with MetSyn results in oxidative stress, endothelial dysfunction, atheroma formation, and inflammation within the atheromatous plaque. Inflammation within the atheromatous plaque causes increased production of metalloproteinases, which results in thinning of the fibrous cap, particularly in the shoulder area, which can lead to plaque rupture or erosion and ACS.

The inflammatory state associated with MetSyn, by worsening endothelial function, allows for increased penetration of the endothelium by LDL particles and monocytes. In the subendothelial space, the trapped LDL particle, particularly the small dense and/or glycosylated LDL particle, is more easily oxidized. These oxidized LDL particles are more easily taken up by macrophages through their scavenger receptor, eventually culminating in the formation of a foam cell. The formation of the foam cell triggers the production of cytokines, which cause inflammation within the plaque. Foam cells also produce growth factors that stimulate proliferation and migration of VSMCs from the media to the intima of the artery, initiating the formation and propagation of atheromatous plaques.

Whether the atheromatous plaque remains stable depends on the amount of inflammation that is occurring within the plaque. The greater the number of white cells within a plaque, the greater the production of cytokines, particularly metalloproteinases, which thin and weaken the fibrous cap. Furthermore, the production of fibrin by the VSMCs, which thickens the fibrous plaque, is suppressed by inflammatory cytokines. Rupture of the fibrous cap, usually at the shoulder area, its weakest point, results in exposure of a surface that stimulates platelet aggregation and coagulation. Clot formation through partial, complete, or embolic obstruction of a coronary artery lumen results in ACS [unstable angina with partial coronary artery occlusion, myocardial infarction (MI) with total coronary occlusion, non-Q wave MI with distal embolization of a clot or sudden death, which in 15% of subjects is the first clinical manifestation of CAD]. Thus, the inflammatory component of MetSyn has a role not only in the development of the atheromatous plaque but also, through plaque rupture, in increases in the frequency of acute and potentially fatal cardiac events.

However, not all coronary artery occlusions are due to plaque rupture. At least 25% of complete or partial coronary artery occlusions occur on areas of plaque where there is endothelial erosion. When compared with plaque rupture, formation of a clot on a endothelial erosion occurs more frequently and is associated with an increased incidence of sudden death. Although the pathogenesis of endothelial erosion is not as well established as that of plaque rupture, endothelial erosion is a more common cause of cardiac events in patients with MetSyn and/or type 2 diabetes.

The importance of inflammation as a component of MetSyn leading to cardiac events was illustrated in the PROVE-IT trial where 3,745 subjects with recent ACS were randomized to 80 mg of the powerful statin atorvastatin or to 40 mg of a weaker statin, pravastatin. Over 3 years, cardiac events greatly favored atorvastatin due to lowering of both LDL cholesterol and hs-CRP, with the greatest reduction in cardiac events occurring when both were lowered to goal. In this study, those who had the elevated hs-CRP were more obese, had higher glucose and triglyceride levels, higher blood pressure, and lower HDL levels. Therefore, the majority of subjects in this study who benefited from the effect of a powerful statin-lowering hs-CRP had MetSyn.

ENDOTHELIAL DYSFUNCTION

MetSyn has been shown to be an independent risk factor for cardiac events even in the presence of other cardiac risk factors such as dyslipidemia, hypertension, and coagulopathy. In the Paris Prospective Study, those nondiabetic subjects with MetSyn who were in the highest quintile for fasting insulin levels (a key marker of MetSyn) had a two- to threefold greater chance of having a cardiac event. In the Quebec Heart Study, fasting insulin levels were shown in nondiabetic males to be an independent risk factor for a cardiac event, with the relative risk being 5.5 for MetSyn compared with 2.5 for an elevated LDL cholesterol level.

One reason that MetSyn is an independent risk factor for cardiac events is its association with endothelial dysfunction. When the endothelium is healthy, nitric oxide production is adequate. Nitric oxide facilitates the artery's ability to vasodilate, provides a "nonstick, nonclot" surface, and suppresses the formation of atheroma by preventing leukocytes from penetrating the endothelium. When the inflammatory state of MetSyn develops, superoxide is produced in excess and nitric oxide is effectively "quenched," which leads to vasoconstriction, thrombosis, and increased formation of atheroma.

A serum marker for endothelial dysfunction, irrespective of the underlying cause, is asymmetric dimethylarginine (ADMA). When MetSyn is treated with a TZD, ADMA levels decrease by 33%. Studies utilizing cardiac positron emission tomography (PET) scans in conjunction with cold pressor testing have shown that the reflex vasodilation that should follow cold-induced vasoconstriction of the coronary arteries is blunted in the presence of MetSyn. Treatment of MetSyn in these subjects with a TZD for 6 months resulted in improved endothelial function and restoration of coronary artery vasodilatation. A study that utilized ultrasound to measure changes in arterial diameter following the release of brachial artery occlusion with a sphygmomanometer showed that reflex vasodilatation associated with MetSyn in nondiabetic subjects was restored with TZD therapy. Therefore, MetSyn is an independent risk factor for cardiac events through its association with endothelial dysfunction.

ALBUMINURIA

The glomerulus functions as an arteriole, and when systemic endothelial dysfunction occurs the glomerulus becomes more permeable to larger molecules, causing excess albumin to leak into the renal tubule. Because not all of this albumin is reabsorbed, excess albumin can be detected in the urine as microalbuminuria (> 30 mg per gram of creatinine) or macroalbuminuria (> 300 mg per gram of creatinine). Therefore, the glomerulus is a "window" for generalized endothelial dysfunction, and the presence of albuminuria correlates well with other tests of endothelial dysfunction. In addition, albuminuria is a marker for atherosclerosis, because when the glomerulus is more permeable to albumin the endothelium becomes more permeable to lipoproteins throughout the vascular tree. Because of this, many studies have found the presence of albuminuria to be an independent risk factor for cardiac events.

In older Danish subjects, microalbuminuria was shown to be a much stronger risk factor than hs-CRP for cardiac events and mortality. In the Islington Diabetes Survey, the presence of microalbuminuria was robustly associated with the presence of diabetes, CAD, and peripheral vascular disease (PAD). However, after 3.6 years, the presence of microalbuminuria at the initial assessment was associated with a 16.5-fold increase in mortality. In the HOPE trial, the presence of microalbuminuria was the best predictor for a CV event, even more so than the presence of preexisting CAD. In the EPIC-Norfolk study, microalbuminuria was independently associated with total and CV mortality. A prospective study of subjects without diabetes, CAD, renal disease, or urinary tract infection showed that not only was microalbuminuria an independent risk factor for cardiac events, but that the presence of microalbuminuria was more than twice as predictive as any of the traditional risk factors for CAD. These findings are probably due to the association of microalbuminuria with endothelial dysfunction and MetSyn.

It should be noted that the lower the albumin-to-creatinine ratio in the urine, the lower the risk of a CV event. Although a cutoff point for the risk of renal disease has been established at 30 mg of albumin per gram of creatinine, for CV risk the threshold is lower—7 mg albumin per gram of creatinine. TZDs, RAAS inhibitors, and carvedilol, a beta blocker that improves inflammation, oxidative stress, and endothelial dysfunction associated with MetSyn, have all been shown to decrease albuminuria in MetSyn patients.

HEART FAILURE AND METABOLIC SYNDROME

A prospective observational study of over 2,000 healthy 50-year-old men who were followed prospectively for 20 years showed that MetSyn was associated with HF. Even after adjusting for other risk factors—cigarette smoking, hypertension, diabetes, BMI, and LVH on an EKG—the risk of HF was increased by two-thirds if MetSyn was judged to be present at baseline. An additional adjustment for the presence of MI increased the risk of HF with MetSyn to 80%.

As discussed in an earlier section, microalbuminuria is a marker for MetSyn. In the Strong Heart Study of Native Americans, even after adjusting for age, gender, BMI, blood pressure, left ventricular mass, and duration of diabetes, microalbuminuria was still a marker of diastolic dysfunction. In the HOPE study, the presence of microalbuminuria was also associated with an increased incidence of HF.

Why are microalbuminuria and MetSyn associated with HF? The most obvious reason is that microalbuminuria is associated with increased permeability of the myocardial microcirculation, which leads to myocardial fibrosis. It is also due to the endothelial dysfunction associated with MetSyn; in the myocardium, vasoconstriction occurs, leading to reperfusion injury and further myocardial fibrosis, which leads to diastolic dysfunction.

Another reason that microalbuminuria is associated with MetSyn and HF is that MetSyn is associated with mitochondrial dysfunction in the myocardiocyte, which leads to accumulation of triglycerides within its cytoplasm. Cardiac magnetic resonance imaging (MRI) studies of subjects with MetSyn and type 2 diabetes have clearly shown that the fat-to-water ratio of the myocardium increases with body weight and decreased levels of glucose tolerance. The metabolism of triglycerides and FFAs leads to the formation of lipotoxic compounds, such as ceramide, which precipitate oxidative stress, which, in turn, leads to increased myocardial apoptosis and further myocardial fibrosis. Therefore, MetSyn is associated with diastolic dysfunction, which is worsened by the presence of LVH and CAD, both of which are also associated with MetSyn.

Therefore, even in the absence of diabetes, MetSyn is a risk factor for HF due to endothelial dysfunction, which causes myocardial fibrosis, LVH, diastolic dysfunction caused by mitochondrial dysfunction and increased myocardial triglycerides, and an increased prevalence of CAD.

Valve calcification, particularly involving the aortic leaflets, is another risk factor for the HF that commonly occurs with longstanding MetSyn. This can lead to valvular dysfunction (stenosis or regurgitation), which may cause or worsen cardiac failure.

As will be discussed in Chapter 4, HF, through increased sympathetic activity and RAAS activation, increases resistance to the action of insulin. The failing heart, to facilitate survival, needs to change its substrate for energy generation from FFA to glucose, which is more efficiently metabolized, therefore decreasing the cardiac workload. Because of resistance to the action of insulin associated with MetSyn, the myocardium cannot take up and utilize glucose, so that myocardial function is not improved. Lowering of insulin resistance with metformin and/or a TZD increases myocardial glucose uptake.

PERIPHERAL ARTERY DISEASE AND METABOLIC SYNDROME

MetSyn, at least in women, has been shown in a prospective study to be associated with a 62% increased risk of future peripheral artery disease (PAD). For each feature of MetSyn that was present, there was a 21% increased risk of PAD. However, these women had elevated levels of hs-CRP and soluble intercellular adhesion molecule-1, which when included in the analysis decreased and negated the association of PAD with MetSyn. Therefore, MetSyn is associated with an increased risk of future PAD, which is largely mediated through the effects of inflammation and damage to the endothelium.

CONCLUSION

Risk factors for cardiac events that are associated with MetSyn include hypertension, LVH, dyslipidemia with small dense LDL and HDL particles, increased platelet aggregation, and decreased fibrinolysis. In addition, MetSyn is an inflammatory state that leads to endothelial dysfunction, of which the presence of microalbuminuria is a marker. MetSyn is also an independent risk factor for HF, myocardial fibrosis, and valvular calcification. Therefore, the presence of MetSyn not only increases the risk of developing diabetes but is also a major CV risk factor.

Chapter 4
Cardiovascular Outcomes of Treating Metabolic Syndrome

LIFESTYLE MODIFICATION AND METABOLIC SYNDROME

Although the manifestations of MetSyn will improve with lifestyle modification (diet, weight loss, and exercise), to date, no objective evidence has shown that it will result in improvements in surrogate markers for atherosclerosis or CV events. Therefore, the evidence for decreases in surrogate markers for atheroma and CV events with therapy of MetSyn is based on randomized controlled trials of pharmacological therapy.

LOWERING OF CARDIAC RISK FACTORS WITH PHARMACOLOGICAL THERAPY

In the UKPDS study, metformin, which improves the manifestations of MetSyn, was shown to decrease cardiac events in obese diabetic subjects. Metformin has also been shown to improve mortality in HF, which is associated with MetSyn. However, studies have shown that the manifestations of MetSyn are improved much more with TZDs.

Clearly the use of TZDs reduces markers of inflammation, microalbuminuria, platelet aggregation, the number of small dense LDL particles, as well as levels of serum insulin, metalloproteinases, triglycerides, and PAI_1. TZDs also increase both total HDL and the number of large HDL particles, insulin sensitivity, and adiponectin levels. Because of improvement in endothelial function with TZDs in subjects with MetSyn, systolic blood pressure decreases by as much as 6 to 8 mm Hg. Although TZDs should not be used as antihypertensives, the reduction in systolic blood pressure is not insignificant, because, particularly in the diabetic patient, small decreases in blood pressure can result in significant decreases in CV events. In the Optimal Therapy of Hypertension (HOT) Study, a 4-mm drop in systolic blood pressure in diabetic subjects resulted in a 51% decrease in CV events. Therefore, even small decreases in systolic blood pressure due to TZD-induced improvements in endothelial function in the subject with MetSyn may be significant.

IMPROVEMENTS IN SURROGATE MARKERS OF ATHEROSCLEROSIS THROUGH PHARMACOLOGICAL TREATMENT

The TZDs have been shown to reduce surrogate markers of atherosclerosis. In a 4-year randomized placebo-controlled study of nondiabetic individuals, rosiglitazone slowed the progression of carotid intima-medial thickening by approximately two-thirds. In another randomized trial that involved 393 individuals with impaired glucose tolerance and a mean BMI of 33 (making this essentially a study of MetSyn individuals), pioglitazone, over the course of 3 years, reduced the rate of progression of carotid intima-medial thickening by 38% annually compared to placebo.

A more accurate method of assessing the volume of atheroma is intravascular ultrasound (IVUS). With coronary angiography, where the coronary arteries are viewed only in two dimensions, significant coronary artery narrowing can be missed. However, IVUS more accurately measures the true atherosclerotic burden, and thus is the current gold standard for the quantitation of the volume of coronary atheroma. In the PERISCOPE study, diabetic patients were randomized to either sulfonylurea glimepiride or the TZD pioglitazone, with coronary artery IVUS being performed at baseline and again after 18 months of treatment. Significant differences favoring pioglitazone were shown for change in coronary atheroma volume (Figure 4.1).

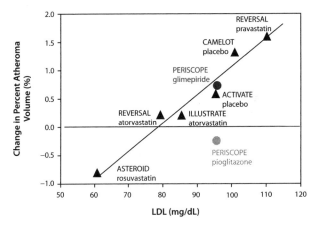

Figure 4.1. PERISCOPE: Comparison to Other Trials

Source: Data in Nissen SE, et al. *JAMA*. 2008;299:1561–1573.

IMPROVEMENT IN CARDIAC EVENTS THROUGH TREATMENT OF
METABOLIC SYNDROME

Because treatment of MetSyn with TZDs results not only in an improvement in cardiac risk factors, but also in a decrease in the volume of coronary and carotid atheroma, TZD therapy should result in decreases in cardiac events. Decreases in cardiac events with rosiglitazone did not occur in the RECORD study, whereas cardiac events decreased significantly with pioglitazone in the PROactive study.

In the PROactive study, uncontrolled type 2 diabetic patients who were judged to be at increased cardiac risk were randomized to the addition of either a placebo or pioglitazone, which was quickly escalated to the maximal dose, to their existing antidiabetic regimen. The primary endpoint of the study was the time from randomization to an acute cardiac event, leg revascularization, or amputation. After 36 months, no significant difference in the primary endpoint was found. However, a predetermined secondary endpoint (MI, death, or stroke) was significantly decreased by 16%. The reason for the difference between these two

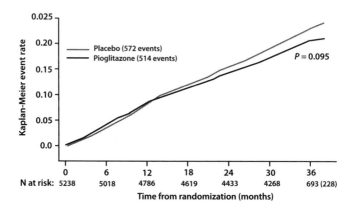

Figure 4.2. PROactive: No Significant Difference in Primary Composite Endpoint*

*All-cause mortality, non-fatal MI (including silent MI), stroke, major leg amputation (above the ankle), acute coronary syndrome, cardiac intervention including CABG or percutaneous coronary intervention, leg revascularization. Pioglitazone vs. placebo: HR: 0.90; 95% CI: 0.80–1.02.

Source: Dormandy J, et al. Secondary prevention of macrovascular events in patients with type 2 diabetes in the PROactive Study (PROspective pioglitAzone Clinical Trial in macroVascular Events): A randomized controlled trial. *The Lancet.* 2005;366(9493):1279–1289. Reprinted with permission from Elsevier.

endpoints was the inclusion of subjects with PAD, who comprised 24% of the participants. Overall, subjects with PAD had higher rates of cardiac events, and the rate of these cardiac events was unaffected by pioglitazone. Eliminating this group from the final analysis resulted in the primary endpoint being very significantly improved with pioglitazone. In addition, in the PROactive study myocardial reinfarction was reduced by 28% and recurrence of the ACS was decreased by 37%. The improvement in reinfarction is consistent with a nonblinded U.S. study, where TZD therapy decreased myocardial reinfarction by 52%. Although the total number of strokes was not decreased with pioglitazone, recurrence of stroke was decreased by 47% (Figures 4.2 and 4.3).

Thus, at least with pioglitazone, improvement in cardiac events by treating MetSyn has been shown. However, the positive results of the PROactive study could also have been due to improvements in other risk factors, such as hemoglobin A1c (HbA1c), which was decreased by 0.5%; or HDL, which was increased by 8.9%; or the systolic blood pressure, which was decreased by 3 mm Hg. In addition, on a retrospective reanalysis of the PROactive study, concurrent use of statins and beta blockers seemed to negate the positive effect of pioglitazone. Realistically, a much larger study would have been needed to show a positive effect of pioglitazone on cardiac events when other cardioprotective drugs, such as statins, beta blockers, and blockers of the renin-angiotensin system, were being utilized.

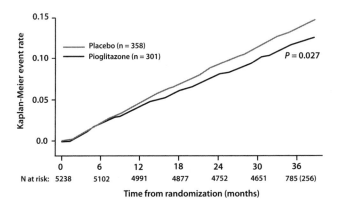

Figure 4.3. PROactive: Significant Difference in Principal Secondary Endpoint*

*Death, MI (excluding silent) or stroke. Pioglitazone vs. placebo: HR: 0.84; 95% CI: 0.72–0.98.

Source: Dormandy J, et al. Secondary prevention of macrovascular events in patients with type 2 diabetes in the PROactive Study (PROspective pioglitAzone Clinical Trial in macroVascular Events): A randomized controlled trial. The Lancet. 2005;366(9493):1279–1289. Reprinted with permission from Elsevier.

HEART FAILURE ASSOCIATED WITH THIAZOLIDINEDIONES

TZDs induce fluid retention by increasing reabsorption of sodium in the very distal renal tubule. Much of the weight gain associated with TZDs may well be due to fluid retention; it has been estimated that up to 10 pounds of fluid can be retained before dependent edema appears. When TZD-induced edema appears, it is dependent edema—the neck veins are not distended and brain natriuretic peptide levels, which are diagnostic of HF, are not elevated.

However, TZDs can increase plasma volume by as much as 6%, and in diabetic patients this may precipitate HF 3 to 5 years before the HF would have presented. Therefore, TZD utilization is a "stress test" for a compromised myocardium and results in earlier utilization of drugs that will improve ventricular function, such as inhibitors of the RAAS and beta blockers.

The reason for a compromised myocardium in the diabetic patient is that, in addition to CAD, 71% of diabetic patients have LVH and 50% to 60% have diabetic cardiomyopathy (see Chapter 3). Because of this "cardiotoxic triad," 42% of patients admitted to the hospital with HF in the United States have diabetes.

Therefore, with the high doses of pioglitazone that were used in the PROactive study, especially in combination with insulin, it is not surprising that there was an increased rate of reported HF. However, because the presence of HF was based on investigator observation, many of these cases could have simply been dependent edema. An increase in hospital admissions with HF would certainly dilute the possibility that the reported HF was largely due to dependent edema.

Therefore, it is significant that with pioglitazone in the PROactive study the rates of both reported HF and admission to hospital with HF were increased. However, it is also very significant that there was no increase in death from HF. In fact, in the PROactive study, if HF occurred in the placebo group, the mortality was higher than if HF occurred in the pioglitazone group.

This data with pioglitazone is in keeping with data derived from Medicare billing, where patients discharged from the hospital with a diagnosis of HF had improved mortality if they were discharged on a TZD and/or metformin. Because these drugs were both contraindicated in HF, discharging HF patients on these drugs could be interpreted as being irresponsible. The major reason that these insulin sensitizers protected these HF patients is that for the failing heart to survive the myocardium needs to change its preferred substrate for the generation of energy from FFA (high-octane fuel) to glucose (low-octane fuel), which will facilitate a decrease in the cardiac workload. Unfortunately, resistance to insulin-induced myocardial uptake of glucose in the presence of MetSyn prevents the myocardium from changing its substrate for metabolism. In addition, in HF, levels of counter-regulatory hormones, such as catecholamines, are elevated, which further increases resistance to the uptake of glucose by the myocardium. The addition of a TZD, or to a lesser extent metformin, reduces insulin resistance and facilitates the uptake of glucose by the myocardium, resulting in a deceased cardiac workload, which, in turn, will improve the likelihood of both the survival of the myocardium and the subject with HF.

Another reason that metformin and TZDs will improve survival is that metformin and TZDs activate the enzyme 5-AMP-activated protein kinase (5-AMPK). Under normal circumstances, in the myocardium 5-AMPK is activated when the cardiomyocytes—either due to decreased adenosine triphosphate (ATP) generation or increased energy demand—have a limited supply of nutrients. 5-AMPK can thus be regarded as a "fuel gauge" and the guardian of cardiac energy, increasing ATP levels by both increasing the generation of ATP and limiting its utilization. In addition, during ischemia and reperfusion it increases glucose uptake and glycolysis and, by limiting apoptosis, decreases reperfusion injury. Thus, TZDs and metformin improve myocardial function and decrease the risk of HF by activating 5-AMPK. Another possible mechanism through which metformin and TZDs improve the outcome for HF patients is that there may be a reversal of "aldosterone escape." With HF, 50% escape RAAS blockade, and this escape correlates well with features of the MetSyn. Improving insulin resistance may reverse the escape from RAAS blockade which is associated with a poor prognosis.

METABOLIC SYNDROME WITH THIAZOLIDINEDIONES, CORONARY ANGIOPLASTY, AND STENTS

MetSyn has been associated with increased restenosis following coronary angioplasty with or without stent placement. Treatment of MetSyn with TZDs, which are anti-inflammatory and antiproliferative, have been shown to decrease restenosis following coronary angioplasty. The advent of drug-eluting stents (DESs) seemed to eliminate the need to use medications other than antiplatelet medications to avoid restenosis. Unfortunately, although DESs have been shown to be superior to bare metal stents, DESs have also been associated with a high rate of late stent thrombosis, which can be a fatal complication. It has been shown that the use of the TZD pioglitazone with a bare metal stent results in less restenosis and a decreased risk of coronary events than when DESs are utilized without the addition of a TZD.

CONCLUSION

Treating MetSyn, especially with TZDs, not only improves cardiac risk factors, but also decreases the formation of atheroma, and, at least with the TZD pioglitazone, decreases the incidence of cardiac events, strokes, and mortality. In addition, the use of TZDs with coronary artery angioplasty and stent placement reduces the rate of restenosis. TZDs can both precipitate HF and reduce mortality due to HF. Metformin's efficacy in treating MetSyn is matched by its less robust effect on decreasing cardiac risk factors, atherosclerosis, and cardiac events.

Chapter 5

Diabetes and the Metabolic Syndrome

RISK OF TYPE 2 DIABETES AND METABOLIC SYNDROME

Approximately 50 million people in the United States have MetSyn; of those, only 35% will develop type 2 diabetes. The other two-thirds avoid the development of diabetes by increasing their production and release of insulin from the pancreatic beta cells to overcome the insulin resistance that is associated with MetSyn. However, failure to develop diabetes does not protect MetSyn subjects from being at increased risk of CV events. Indeed, in the Nurses' Health Study those who developed diabetes had a greater risk of MI or stroke prior to being diagnosed with diabetes than they had following the diagnosis of diabetes.

THE NATURAL HISTORY OF THE DEVELOPMENT OF DIABETES WITH METABOLIC SYNDROME

The 30% to 40% of MetSyn patients who develop diabetes initially increase their production and release of insulin to overcome the insulin resistance associated with MetSyn but eventually reach a point where the pancreatic beta cells cannot continue to secrete these excessive amounts of insulin. When this occurs, insulin secretion gradually decreases until diabetes develops. Prior to this, as insulin secretion decreases there is a period of variable length during which impaired glucose intolerance is present. At the glucose-intolerance stage, the insulin secretory capacity of the pancreatic beta cells is adequate to maintain fasting and preprandial glucose levels in the normal range but is unable to generate an insulin spike adequate to maintain the postprandial glucose levels in a normal healthy range.

With the glucose tolerance test, impaired glucose tolerance is defined as a 2-hour glucose of between 140 and 200 mg/dL; a 2-hour level in excess of 200 mg/dL is diagnostic for diabetes, irrespective of the fasting glucose. Additionally, two fasting glucoses of above 126 mg/dL, or a random glucose of over 200 mg/dL accompanied by symptoms of hyperglycemia, is diagnostic for diabetes. In addition, diabetes may now be diagnosed with an HbA1c above 6.5%.

Insulin production and release begins to diminish as early as 12 years before type 2 diabetes is diagnosed. By the time diabetes is diagnosed, the insulin-producing beta cells are functioning at a level of 50% or less of the capacity at which these cells were functioning before the beta cells became dysfunctional. Six years after the diagnosis of diabetes the beta cells are functioning at 25% of capacity, and after 10 years from type 2 diabetes diagnosis at 10% of capacity, and by this time most patients need insulin.

The relentless decline in beta cell function is not affected by lifestyle changes or therapy with sulfonylureas, insulin, or metformin. Injectable incretin mimetics, such as exenatide-4 or liraglutide and TZDs, are the only therapies that have been shown to decelerate the decline in or even improve beta cell function.

Gastric bypass surgery is a cure for type 2 diabetes even before weight loss occurs, because rapid gastric emptying increases the production of the incretin, glucagon-like peptide (GLP_1), from the K cells of the terminal ileum. The increased levels of GLP_1 improve beta cell function so that 70% to 80% of cases of type 2 diabetes are cured following gastric bypass surgery. The incretin mimetics increase GLP_1 activity, to a level that is enough to significantly improve beta cell function but not to the level obtained with gastric bypass surgery. Dipeptyl peptidase-4 (DPP-4) inhibitors, which suppress the activity of the enzyme DPP-4, which rapidly metabolizes GLP_1, also increase GLP_1 levels. However, the increased GLP_1 levels that occur with DPP-4 inhibition are much lower than those achieved with gastric bypass surgery or incretin mimetics and, to date, at least in humans, have not been shown to improve beta cell function.

ETIOLOGY AND PATHOPHYSIOLOGY OF TYPE 2 DIABETES

Why beta cell function declines in some patients and not in others with MetSyn is unknown. To solve the problem would require biopsies of the pancreas in a living person, which is neither practical nor ethical. However, autopsy studies have clearly shown that the beta cell volume is decreased in diabetic subjects and that beta cell replication is not decreased, and indeed may be increased, especially in those who are obese. The major mechanism that is responsible for decreasing beta cell volume and function is apoptosis (programmed cell death), which is accelerated in both the thin and obese type 2 diabetic subjects. Therefore, the decreased beta cell mass and insulin production from the diabetic beta cells is due to beta cell apoptosis and not to decreased formation of new beta cells. Although drugs that increase beta cell proliferation may be helpful in preserving beta cell function, only drugs that can also decelerate beta cell apoptosis will result in a meaningful improvement in beta cell function (Figure 5.1).

With decreased beta cell function, the ratio of proinsulin (the precursor of insulin) to insulin is elevated, illustrating that reduced beta cell capacity causes insulin to be released prematurely. In the Women's Health Study, normoglycemic subjects who were in the top quartile of the proinsulin-to-insulin ratio had a 10-fold increased risk of developing type 2 diabetes.

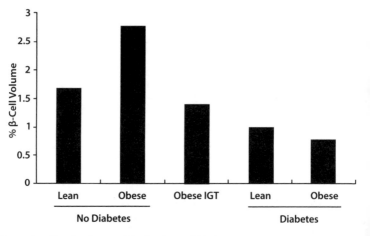

Figure 5.1. β-Cell Volume with Obesity and Diabetes

Source: Butler A, et al. β-cell deficit and increased β-cell apoptosis in humans with type 2 diabetes. *Diabetes.* 2003;52:102–110.

The etiology of the decline in beta cell function in type 2 diabetes is related to four risk factors:

1. **Glucotoxicty.** With rising glucose levels, the release of insulin from the beta cell is decreased, and correction of hyperglycemia results not only in improved insulin sensitivity in the myocytes, adipocytes, and hepatocytes but also in improved insulin release from the pancreatic beta cells. An extreme example of this is the patient who is admitted to hospital with hyperosmolar coma due to extremely high glucose levels. Following correction of the hyperglycemia, possible due to repletion of the anti-oxidant NAPDH, insulin resistance decreases and insulin secretion increases, so that many of these patients at the time of discharge from the hospital are easily and well controlled on oral agents. In addition, chronic glucotoxicity, especially when combined with sulfonylurea therapy, decreases NAPDH levels and accelerates the decline in beta cell function.

2. **Amyloid deposition.** Amyloid is an inflammatory protein that is cosecreted with insulin. Especially in the later stages of type 2 diabetes, amyloid precipitates due to the presence of toxic amyloid oligomers and is deposited in the beta cells, where it interferes with insulin secretion and release. Mice, unlike humans, do not deposit amyloid in the pancreatic beta cells. Knockout mice given the human gene for amyloid deposition will only deposit amyloid in the pancreatic beta cells when exposed to a high-fat diet, and amyloid deposition can be reduced, or even prevented, with the use of a

TZD. Therefore, amyloid deposition is probably, but has not been proven to be, related to MetSyn. Toxic oligomers induce stress in the endoplasmic reticulum and disrupt cell coupling, leading to apoptosis.

3. **Inflammation.** Autopsy studies have shown increased amounts of proinflammatory cytokines in the pancreatic beta cells of type 2 diabetic patients and that the number of macrophages per islet cell is five times higher in diabetic than in the nondiabetic subjects. The macrophages are also centrally located in the diabetic subject, whereas in the nondiabetic they are more peripherally located. The presence of these macrophages leads to increased cytokine levels, which, in turn, leads to oxidative stress that accelerates beta cell apoptosis.

4. **Lipotoxicity.** In most cells of the body, aging and declining mitochondrial function cause the triglyceride content of the cytoplasm to increase. Human autopsy studies have shown that with aging the cells of the pancreatic duct and the pancreatic alpha cells contain more lipid, but that pancreatic beta cells accumulate twice as much cytoplasmic lipid as these cells. This suggests that mitochondrial function decreases more in pancreatic beta cells than other cells with aging and that the beta cells are more vulnerable to the mitochondrial dysfunction associated with MetSyn.

BETA CELL DAMAGE FROM LIPOTOXICITY ASSOCIATED WITH METABOLIC SYNDROME

Why does MetSyn cause more fat to accumulate in the cytoplasm of the pancreatic beta cell? MetSyn is associated with increased cytoplasmic fat in muscle, the liver, and the myocardium as well as in the pancreatic beta cells due to both genetic and aging factors. Genetically, there is a decrease in mitochondrial oxidative phosphorylation of FFAs, so that FFAs cannot enter the mitochondria for oxidation and are stored as triglycerides in the cytoplasm. With aging, mitochondrial function decreases further, leading to greater accumulation of cytoplasmic lipid. MetSyn, probably due to a deficiency of adiponectin, is also associated with increased lipolysis of peritoneal adipocytes and hepatic fat, which increases serum FFA levels, leading to an even greater increase in beta cell cytoplasmic triglyceride.

Lipolysis of cytoplasmic triglyceride leads to increased cytoplasmic FFA levels and its metabolites acyl-CoA, diaglycerol, and ceramide. Although all of these metabolites have an effect on apoptosis, ceramide has the greatest effect. Ceramide, by stimulating the activity of nitric oxide synthase, leads to the generation of excessive and toxic levels of nitric oxide. This nitric oxide combines with superoxide to form peroxynitrite, which accelerates beta cell apoptosis.

With accelerated beta cell apoptosis, the lifespan of the beta cell is decreased, and the loss of beta cells mass associated with the accelerated apoptosis is inadequately compensated for by an increased formation of new beta cells from stem cells in the pancreatic duct. Therefore, over time the pancreatic beta cell mass shrinks and a relative insulin deficiency develops.

ANIMAL STUDIES SHOWING IMPROVED BETA CELL FUNCTION WITH THERAPY OF METABOLIC SYNDROME

In animal studies, through removal of fat from the pancreatic beta cell, TZDs have been shown to suppress apoptosis and improve beta cell function. Similarly, incretin mimetics and gastric bypass surgery, both of which increase GLP_1 activity, suppress apoptosis and increase proliferation of the beta cells. These therapies have been shown to improve beta cell function. In addition, animal, but not human, studies have shown that DPP-4 inhibitors, which to a lesser extent increase circulating GLP_1 levels, restore normoglycemia in 27% of animals. In the same animals, if the DPP-4 inhibitor is combined with a proton-pump inhibitor, which by elevating gastrin levels also increases the beta cell mass, normoglycemia was restored in 81% of animals.

HUMAN STUDIES SHOWING IMPROVED BETA CELL FUNCTION WITH THERAPY OF METABOLIC SYNDROME

Studies with TZDs that have shown superior sustained glycemic control compared with other oral antidiabetic agents or that have prevented the development of diabetes or delayed the need to use insulin injections will be reviewed in Chapter 6. The evidence with incretin mimetics and DPP-4 inhibitors is more limited than that found in animal studies, where induction of insulin gene transcription and increased insulin biosynthesis have been verified. A 1-year study comparing the effects of the incretin mimetic exenatide (GLP_1 receptor stimulator) and the long-acting insulin glargine in type 2 diabetic patients showed that with both glucose and arginine stimulation (measures of functional and maximal beta cell function, respectively) endogenous insulin production with exenatide was 2.6-fold greater than that with the long-acting insulin.

Similarly, the incretin mimetic liraglutide (victoza) in human studies has been shown to restore first phase insulin release, improve second phase insulin release, increase C-peptide levels, and decrease the ratio of proinsulin to insulin.

CONCLUSION

Treatment of type 2 diabetes should, wherever possible, be directed at improving or preserving beta cell function. Therapies that preserve beta cell function should be used in preference to therapies that do not improve or that in the long-term may even worsen beta cell function. This means that TZDs and incretin mimetics should be utilized early in the course of type 2 diabetes when the potential to maximize beta cell function is at its zenith, not at a later stage when beta cell function is approaching its nadir and the potential for salvaging substantial pancreatic beta cells secretory function is diminished. Therefore, in new-onset diabetes, a combination of a TZD and an incretin mimetic should produce the best long-term results, because preservation of beta cell function results not only in better glycemic control but also in fewer long-term diabetic complications.

Chapter 6

Metabolic Outcomes Resulting from the Treatment of the Metabolic Syndrome

INTRODUCTION

The major metabolic outcomes from treating MetSyn are the prevention of diabetes, improvement in the control of existing diabetes, controlling post-prandial glucose, and delay in the need to use insulin injections in the type 2 diabetic patient.

LIFESTYLE MODIFICATION

The effect of lifestyle modification (decreased calorie intake, weight loss, and increased physical activity) has been clearly shown to at least delay, and in many cases avoid, the development of diabetes. In the Finnish Diabetes Prevention study, obese, middle-aged subjects with impaired glucose tolerance were randomized to intensive lifestyle intervention or to a control group. Intensive lifestyle therapy, after a median of 3 years, reduced the development of type 2 diabetes by 43%. After 7 years—4 years after the end of the study—this group still showed a 36% reduction in the development of diabetes.

The Indian Diabetes Prevention Program (IDPP) showed that subjects with impaired glucose tolerance who were randomized to lifestyle therapy (a 7% loss of body weight and 150 minutes of exercise per week) were 58% less likely to progress to type 2 diabetes than was the control group over the course of the 3-year study. The Da Qing IGT and Diabetes study included 577 subjects with impaired glucose tolerance who were randomized to diet alone, exercise alone, or diet and exercise for 5 years. This resulted in reductions in the development of diabetes by 31% with diet, 46% with exercise, and 42% with both diet and exercise, suggesting that exercise is the most effective tool in the prevention of type 2 diabetes.

In another study, Australian Aborigines who were city dwellers but had been raised in their native environment returned to their native "hunter-gatherer" lifestyle for 3 weeks.

During these 3 weeks, the subjects' exercise and protein intake increased and fat intake decreased. After 3 weeks, body weight remained unchanged but glucose tolerance improved and insulin levels were reduced, indicating improvements in both insulin resistance and MetSyn from lifestyle modification.

In the Toranomon study, Japanese males with impaired glucose tolerance who were treated with lifestyle therapy had a 67.4% reduction in conversion to diabetes compared with the control group, largely due to greater weight loss (0.39 versus 2.12 kg). In the United States, the Diabetes Prevention Trial (DPT) found that lifestyle modification reduced progression from impaired glucose tolerance to type 2 diabetes by 58% over the course of the 3-year study.

PHARMACOLOGICAL INTERVENTION

Another arm of the DPT study showed that metformin reduced progression from impaired glucose tolerance to type 2 diabetes by 31%, but that metformin was less effective than lifestyle change, especially in older subjects. Similarly, the IDPP found that metformin reduced progression to type 2 diabetes by 26.4%. Therefore, metformin therapy can, by its effect on appetite, food intake, and weight loss, improve both insulin resistance and MetSyn and, by decreasing hepatic glucose production, prevent or delay the development of type 2 diabetes.

A more effective MetSyn therapy is the utilization of TZDs. In addition to lowering insulin resistance, these agents also improve beta cell function. In the Troglitazone in Prevention of Diabetes (TRIPOD) study, development of diabetes was decreased by 55% with troglitazone in a high-risk group of Hispanic subjects with a history of gestational diabetes. In the DPT, troglitazone was used for only an average of 0.9 years and then withdrawn because of hepatotoxicity. However, during the time that troglitazone was utilized the development of diabetes was decreased by 75%, which was a greater than that which occurred with metformin or lifestyle modification during that time period. In the Diabetes Reduction Assessment with ramipril and rosiglitazone medication (DREAM) trial, rosiglitazone decreased the development of diabetes in patients with impaired glucose tolerance by 55%. More impressive, in the Actos Now for Prevention of Diabetes (ACT NOW) trial, pioglitazone in patients with impaired glucose tolerance reduced the development of diabetes by 81%.

With recent-onset diabetes in the A Diabetes Outcome Progression Trial (ADOPT) trial, the longevity of the effectiveness of rosiglitazone monotherapy was greater than that of glyburide or metformin. Therefore, the time to utilization of insulin should be increased with TZDs and exceed that of both glyburide and metformin.

DELAYING THE NEED TO USE INSULIN

TZDs prolong the life of the beta cell by removing fat from the cytoplasm of the beta cell, which decreases both inflammation and oxidative stress, and by suppressing beta cell apoptosis. As a result, TZD therapy for patients with established diabetes improves glycemic control and delays or even avoids the need to initiate insulin therapy.

When the first TZD, troglitazone, became available, patients who were failing a combination of metformin and a sulfonylurea and who would have needed the addition of insulin to regain glycemic control were instead placed on triple oral therapy through the addition of troglitazone, and over the next 6 months HbA1c levels returned to the therapeutic range. At that time it was thought that this was only a temporary remission from the need to use insulin therapy and that insulin therapy would have to be initiated within a few months. However, after 6 years 51% of these patients still had an HbA1c below 7.0% and their HbA1c was superior to the HbA1c of those who had progressed to insulin therapy. In addition, and in spite of this inferior glycemic control, the group on insulin gained significantly more weight.

A later prospective study showed that those subjects who had maintained glycemic control had improved beta cell function. Another group of patients failing a metformin and sulfonylurea regimen were randomized to either the addition of the TZD rosiglitazone or to the addition of insulin. After 6 months, glycemic control improved equally in both groups, but those on rosiglitazone had improved beta cell function, as evidenced by a decreased proinsulin-to-insulin ratio and an increased disposition index. The first phase insulin response, the loss of which occurs early in the course of type 2 diabetes, returned with rosiglitazone but not with insulin.

The return of first-phase insulin release lowers post-prandial glucose. Lowering of post-prandial glugose is the most important glycemic factor in lowering the HbA1c if the HbA1c is 7.5% or below. However, lowering of post-prandial glucose with a TZD (but not with metformin, DPP4 inhibitors, sulfonylureas, or insulins) is associated with lowering of post-prandial triglycerides. As a result, control of post-prandial dysmetabolism (glucose and triglycerides) results in a decrease in formation of atheroma and cardiac events.

In multiple population studies, post-prandial glucose levels have been associated with decreased coronary heart disease and mortality. The HOORN, DECODE, Honolulu Whitehall, Helsinki Policemen, and Paris Prospective studies, which included our 45,000 subjects, the two-hour glucose was associated with increased cardiac events and mortality.

A study of non-diabetic females with normal glucose tolerance and coronary angiography at baseline and after three years. The lower the two-hour glucose tolerance test then the lower was the increase in the volume of coronary atheroma. Indeed, if the two-hour glucose was below 86 mg/dl, there was regression of coronary atheroma volume. Therefore, even within the normal range, the higher the post-prandial glucose, the greater is the rate of atheroma formation.

The DECODE study showed that mortality could not be predicted from the fasting glucose levels but could be predicted from the post-prandial glucose levels, which were, shown to be an independent risk factor for mortality.

The STOP-NIDDM study, a blinded study of 1429 individuals with impaired glucose tolerance assessed whether the alfa-glucosidase inhibitor could slow progression to type 2 diabetes. While conversion to diabetes was significantly reduced by 25%, the relative risk of a cardiovascular event was reduced by 49%. Subsequently, the phase 3 studies of acarbose were reexamined for cardiovascular events and it was found that comared with placebo and other diabetic medications, the risk of having a myocardial infarct was decreased by 64% and the risk of any cardiovascular event decreased by 35% with acarbose (Table 6.1). Additionally, acarbose decreased carotid infima-medial thickening by 50%, which reversed when acarbose

Table 6.1. Acarbose and Cardiac Outcomes

Study	Numbers	Result
STOP-NIDDM	1429 IGT	25% RR diabetes 49% RR CVD events 2.5% AR CVD events
Type 2 studies Placebo vs. Acarbose	2230 subjects with diabetes in 7 studies	MI HR 0.36* CVE HR 0.65
IMT		Reduced 50%

Source: Chiasson JL. *Lancet*. 2002;359:20272–20277; Chiasson JL. *JAMA*. 2003;290:486–494; Hanefeldt M. *Stroke*. 2004;35:1073–1078.

was discontinued. Therefore, a benefit of the return of first phase insulin response is lowering of cardiac events. DPP4 inhibitors and incretin mimetics also restore the first phase insulin response and also suppress glucagon production, which further decreases post-prandial glucose elevations.

Therefore, treating the manifestations of MetSyn will not only improve insulin resistance but will also improve beta cell function and delay and possibly avoid altogether the need for insulin therapy.

CONCLUSION

Treating MetSyn with lifestyle changes and TZDs results in decreases in the development of type 2 diabetes, improved glycemic control with established type 2 diabetes, and a delay in the need to utilize insulin. In addition, lowering insulin resistance improves post-prandial glucose and lipid levels, which should decrease cardiac events.

Chapter 7

Metabolic Syndrome and the Liver

NONALCOHOLIC FATTY LIVER DISEASE

Nonalcoholic fatty liver disease (NAFLD) encompasses the conditions of nonalcoholic steatosis, nonalcoholic steatohepatitis (NASH), NASH-cirrhosis, and hepatocellular carcinoma in patients with NASH cirrhosis.

NAFLD is the most common liver disease in the United States, with an estimated prevalence of 34% in adults, 9.6% in children, and 38% in obese children. On ultrasound, as many as 78% of patients with type 2 diabetes have hepatic fat.

NAFLD is associated with all of the characteristics of MetSyn. Insulin and C-peptide levels are increased in nondiabetic NASH patients and in patients with type 2 diabetes. Hepatic fat content is the best predictor of the amount of insulin needed to lower the serum glucose. In fact, it has been suggested that peritoneal fat is an "innocent bystander" and that the real "culprit" responsible for the features of MetSyn is hepatic fat. A study comparing obese subjects with the same visceral fat volume showed that the volume of hepatic fat but not peritoneal fat was proportional to the markers of MetSyn.

Table 7.1. Insulin Resistance and Non-Alcoholic Fatty Liver Disease

	NAFLD (N = 46)	Controls (N = 92)
W/H ratio	0.89*	0.84
HDL (mg/dL)	46.4*	54.2
Triglyceride (mg/dL)	223*	125
FBG (mg/dL)	94*	90
Fasting insulin (µU/mL)	14.4*	8.4
C-peptide (pmol/mL)	3.5*	1.9

* p = .001.

NAFLD develops due to increased production of FFAs, which further decreases the function of the hepatocyte mitochondria, which are already compromised by genetic and age-related defects. The combination of elevated FFAs and mitochondrial dysfunction causes fat to accumulate in the liver. In addition, a correlation exists between low adiponectin levels and hepatic fat, and it is believed that adiponectin deficiency may be a prime factor in the development of NAFLD.

NONALCOHOLIC STEATOHEPATITIS

The sinister form of NAFLD is NASH, which is characterized by perisinusoidal inflammation, hepatic necrosis, and hepatocyte regeneration. When these changes result in fibrosis and alteration of hepatic architecture, cirrhosis, portal hypertension, and end-stage liver disease occur. In the United States, NASH is the most common cause of nonalcoholic liver failure. Why only 25% of NAFLD cases progress to NASH is not known, but it may be related to the severity of MetSyn, because those who advance to NASH have more severe manifestations of MetSyn (i.e., they are more obese, have lower adiponectin levels, are more likely to have type 2 diabetes, and have more hepatic fat). An increase in hepatic fat content results in an increased production of adipocytokines, such as TNF-α, which may well be the principle inflammatory cytokine associated with the development of NASH.

Accumulation of hepatic fat also results in induction of cytochromes P-450, 4A, and E, which results in increased cytokine production, as well as increased lipid peroxidation, leading to increased aldehyde production. Excess hepatic aldehyde production accelerates apoptosis of the hepatocyte as well as hepatic necrosis and scarring.

Therefore, for NASH to develop a "double hit" must occur. The first insult is the accumulation of hepatic fat; the second is the excess production of adipocytokines and aldehyde. The pathophysiological features of NASH are hepatocyte injury, which clinically is associated in most cases with elevation of transaminases and the pathological ballooning degeneration of hepatocytes, the presence of Mallory hyaline bodies, and infiltration by polymorphonuclear leukocytes. The presence of these features predicts a 25% chance (compared with a 3% chance with NAFLD) of developing cirrhosis as well as a 50% 10-year mortality resulting from either the development of hepatic failure or hepatocellular carcinoma.

NONALCOHOLIC STEATOHEPATITIS IN COMBINATION WITH HEPATITIS C VIRUS

Because NAFLD and hepatitis C virus (HCV) infection are the most common liver diseases in the Western hemisphere, and because HCV infection is more common in type 2 diabetes, it is not surprising that these two conditions often coexist. Hepatic steatosis is present in 50% of HCV-infected subjects, and the combination of steatosis and HCV infection leads to increased fibrosis and an increased likelihood of not responding to antiviral therapy.

IMPROVING NASH BY TREATING METABOLIC SYNDROME

Dietary therapy with a modest weight loss [7 lb (3.2 kg)] in NASH patients results only in a decrease in transaminase levels without an improvement in steatosis or the pathophysiological features of NASH. However, significant weight loss with bariatric surgery results not only in significant decreases in transaminase levels but also decreased steatosis and improvements in the histological features of NASH.

Thus, meaningful weight loss can result in significant reductions in the manifestations of MetSyn and improvements in both NAFLD and NASH. Therefore, pharmaceutically treating MetSyn should result in similar or even greater improvements. Although decreasing hepatic fat, metformin, with its weaker effects on MetSyn, has not been shown to improve the histological features of NASH. In contrast, the TZDs, with their more substantial beneficial effects on MetSyn, result not only in decreased transaminases and hepatic fat, but also in an improvement in hepatic histology, as has been shown in three nonrandomized trials of TZD therapy in hepatic steatohepatitis. More definitive evidence of the effects of TZDs on NASH comes from a placebo-controlled randomized trial that showed that the TZD pioglitazone significantly reduced transaminases, steatosis, inflammation, and hepatic necrosis. In addition, a trend toward reduced hepatic fibrosis was found, matching the findings of animal studies where pioglitazone prevented the activation of stellate cells, which mediate hepatic fibrosis.

Therefore, therapy of MetSyn with TZDs to reduce hepatic fat and hepatic inflammation would seem to be an ideal therapy for preventing the progression of NAFLD to NASH and NASH to end-stage liver disease and hepatic carcinoma.

CONCLUSION

In conclusion, MetSyn is associated with NAFLD, NASH, hepatic cirrhosis, and hepatocellular carcinoma. The mechanism by which hepatic damage occurs is through the production of adipocytokines and aldehydes. Therapy of MetSyn with bariatric–surgery-induced weight loss or TZD therapy can prevent, and even reverse, the progress of MetSyn and NAFD.

Chapter 8

Genitourinary Manifestations of Metabolic Syndrome

POLYCYSTIC OVARIAN SYNDROME

Polycystic ovarian syndrome (PCOS) affects approximately 8% of females in the reproductive age group. It is grossly underdiagnosed and is often associated with MetSyn in premenopausal females.

PATHOGENESIS OF POLYCYSTIC OVARIAN SYNDROME

With MetSyn, muscle, fat, and hepatic tissue become resistant to insulin, and thus insulin levels are increased. High insulin levels acting through the hypothalamus increase the release of both luteinizing hormone releasing hormone (LHRH) from the hypothalamus and luteinizing hormone (LH) from the pituitary gland. Indeed, one of the features of PCOS is a reversal of the ratio of LH to follicular-stimulating hormone (FSH). FSH is a gonadotrophin produced by the pituitary gland, and FSH levels normally exceed those of LH. The presence of excess LH stimulates both ovarian androgenesis and the release of androgens from the ovaries.

Hyperinsulinemia directly stimulates excessive production of androgens from both the ovaries and the zona fasciculata of the cortex of the adrenal glands. Increased insulin levels acting on the liver increase the production of both insulin-like growth factor 1 (IGF_1) and its binding protein ($IGFBP_1$). IGF_1 also stimulates the production of androgens from both the adrenal cortex and the ovary. Elevated insulin levels also suppress hepatic production of sex hormone-binding globulin (SHBG), which increases the levels of unbound, and therefore active, plasma androgens. Clinically, this can be detected by an elevated free testosterone level, and it is the free and not the bound testosterone that accounts for the clinical manifestations of hyperandrogenemia. Indeed, due to decreased SHBG, total testosterone levels are often normal, or even low normal, in PCOS (Figure 8.1).

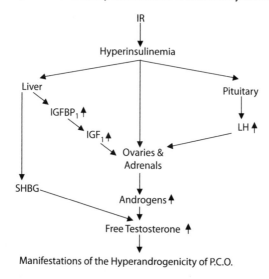

Manifestations of the Hyperandrogenicity of P.C.O.

Figure 8.1. Mechanism for IR in PCOS

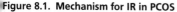

CLINICAL MANIFESTATIONS OF POLYCYSTIC OVARIAN SYNDROME

Because of increased levels of testosterone within the ovary, ovulation is suppressed; additionally, hyperinsulinemia suppresses follicular development. Decreased follicular development and suppression of ovulation not only leads to infertility, but also to menstrual disturbances, including amenorrhea.

Systemically, the effects of elevated free testosterone depend on the degree of elevation. A mild elevation of free testosterone will result in hirsutism and acne. Higher free testosterone levels will lead to temporal recession of the hair line, crown baldness, and clitoromegaly. Interestingly, in males it has been suggested that premature and severe loss of scalp hair is associated with MetSyn. Indeed, epidemiological studies have associated this androgenic alopecia with insulin resistance, as assessed by the homeostasis model assessment of insulin resistance, hypertension, and premature CAD. In women, very high free testosterone levels may manifest as an increase in muscle mass, and even in the development of a male body habitus and male behavior.

Table 8.1. Manifestations of the Hyperandrogenicity of PCOS

1. Ovary
   - Anovulation
   - Menstrual Disturbance
   - Infertility
2. Systemic
   - Hirsutism
   - Acne
   - Cliteromegaly
   - Temporal Recession
   - Crown Baldness
   - Increased Muscle Bulk
   - Male Body Habitus
   - Male Behavior

The long-term clinical features of PCOS include a high likelihood of diabetes and CV disease. By age 50, at least 40% of women with PCOS will have been diagnosed with type 2 diabetes, and following the menopause there is a 7.5-fold increase in the incidence of MI. Thus, recognition of PCOS prior to menopause hastens recognition of a group of women who are at high risk of CV events and have an increased mortality. Aggressive therapy of CV risk factors and treatment of the MetSyn itself is advisable before menopause and is essential after menopause (Table 8.1).

TREATMENT OF POLYCYSTIC OVARIAN SYNDROME

Studies focusing on diet, exercise, and weight loss, which improve resistance to the action of insulin and decrease insulin levels, and the use of diazoxide, which suppresses insulin release from the pancreas, have all shown decreases in serum androgen levels in women with PCO syndrome. In addition, D-chiro-inosotol, which activates enzymes that accelerate the oxidative and nonoxidative metabolism of glucose and lower serum insulin levels, lowered total androgen (including adrenal androgens) and free testosterone level while increasing SHBG levels when utilized in women with PCOS. In a group of women with PCOS, use of D-chiro-inosotol resulted in an ovulation rate of 77.3%, compared with 27.3% in the placebo group.

Similarly, treating MetSyn in these patients with metformin and TZDs has been associated with ovulation, return of menses, and restoration of fertility. Metformin, because it is safe to use during pregnancy, has been more widely studied than TZDs in PCOS women of childbearing age.

A 1994 observational study of women with PCOS and oligomenorrhea in South America showed that metformin lowered testosterone and LH levels and reduced body weight. In addition, menses returned in 55% of the subjects, and pregnancy was achieved in 10%. In the United States, a randomized, placebo-controlled, blinded study of obese women with PCOS confirmed that lowering serum insulin levels with metformin ameliorated hyperandrogenemia. It was later shown that the ovulatory response to the estrogen receptor-blocker clomiphene could be increased by decreasing insulin levels with metformin. However, a later study comparing clomiphene with metformin and a combination of metformin and clomiphene showed that clomiphene was superior in achieving live births in infertile women with PCOS. Unfortunately, that study was performed with extended-release metformin, which is probably not as effective as standard metformin in lowering insulin and androgen levels.

Several studies on the use of the TZD troglitazone in women with PCOS showed significantly greater decreases in free testosterone, adrenal-derived testosterone, estrogen, and insulin levels with troglitazone compared to metformin. Studies of the TZD rosiglitazone have also shown it to be more effective than metformin in the obese PCOS population. Ovulation also occurred more often when rosiglitazone was combined with clomiphene than when the clomiphene was combined with metformin. Similarly, the TZD pioglitazone has been shown to ameliorate the hyperandrogenic activity of the ovary and adrenal glands that occurs in patients with PCOS with the decreases in androgen levels being at least as great as those that occurred with metformin. Overall, although more data exist with metformin, TZDs seem to be more effective than metformin in lowering androgen levels and inducing ovulation.

OVARIAN MANIFESTATIONS OF METABOLIC SYNDROME
OUTSIDE THE FERTILE YEARS

Premature pubarche is a condition whereby girls younger than age 8 develop axillary and pubic hair before the presence of breast development or menstruation; premature pubarche associated with MetSyn. In girls, the physiological sequence of events in sexual development thelarche (breast development), pubarche (development of axillary and pubic hair), and then menarche (start of menstruation). With premature pubarche, thelarche and menarche occur at the normal times and both are preceded by pubarche. Another name for pubarche adrenarche, because the production of androgens from the zona reticulata of the adrenal cortex is responsible for the development of pubic and axillary hair. Physiologically, the zona reticulata is active in utero, but it is inactive between birth and pubarche.

Premature pubarche is associated with the manifestations of MetSyn occurring in conjunction with obesity, lipid abnormalities, and high serum insulin levels. As with PCOS, high insulin levels stimulate the zona reticulata to produce unphysiological amounts of adrenal androgens. Not surprisingly, following puberty these children exhibit manifestations of MetSyn, including increases in the prevalence of PCOS, type 2 diabetes, and CV disease.

In the postmenopausal female, serum testosterone levels usually decrease. However, in some women, due to retained thecal cells that are stimulated by the high gonadotrophin (FSH and LH) levels caused by decreased ovarian estrogen production and impaired activity of the aromatases enzyme, which converts testosterone to estrogen, increased testosterone levels can be present for up to 10 years after the menopause. In addition, when MetSyn is present, high serum insulin levels can cause an additional increase in the production of adrenal and ovarian androgens. If a postmenopausal female presents with clinical features of hyperandrogenemia, this non-neoplastic ovarian hypersecretion of androgens can, in conjunction with abdominal and pelvic imaging, be differentiated from the hyperandrogenemia caused by an adrenal or an ovarian tumor through the ability of high-dose metformin to suppress testosterone levels. By decreasing insulin levels, metformin will decrease serum testosterone by 40% and often bring the testosterone levels back down into the normal range. If the hyperandrogenemia is due to a tumor, suppression of testosterone levels will not occur with the "metformin suppression test."

PREECLAMPTIC TOXEMIA AND PREGNANCY

Compared with controls, women with preeclamptic toxemia or pregnancy-induced hypertension have a 2.7-fold increase in having features of the MetSyn, and for every feature of MetSyn the odds of developing preeclamptic toxemia are increased by 39%. The odds of developing preeclamptic toxemia are also increased fourfold if an elevated hs-CRP level is present.

In another group of women who had had preeclamptic toxemia during pregnancy 6 months after delivery the women had significantly increased systolic blood pressure, waist circumference, and triglyceride levels and lower HDL levels. When studied using the hyperinsulinemic clamp technique, these women were also shown to have a lower sensitivity to the action of insulin. Preeclamptic toxemia is less likely to recur in a subsequent pregnancy, but in a group of women in whom preeclamptic toxemia occurred more than once the presence of a low HDL cholesterol level was shown to be a risk factor for its development in a subsequent pregnancy. In addition, women with PCOS have a higher incidence of preeclamptic toxemia and, like PCOS, preeclampsia is associated with hyperandrogenemia.

A logical hypothesis to explain the association of MetSyn with preeclamptic toxemia is that both are associated with endothelial dysfunction. The classical triad that occurs with preeclamptic toxemia is hypertension, proteinuria, and edema, all of which are associated with endothelial dysfunction. In addition, placental insufficiency, which is also a feature of preeclamptic toxemia, could be caused by endothelial dysfunction, because women with a history of preeclampsia have been shown to have decreased reflex vasodilatation.

TESTICULAR MANIFESTATIONS OF METABOLIC SYNDROME

Hypogonadotrophic hypogonadism (HH) is associated with MetSyn, and more than one-third to one-half of men with type 2 diabetes have low testosterone levels accompanied by low gonadotrophin (FSH and LH) levels, indicating that the problem is not at the level of the testes but rather at the level of the anterior pituitary gland and/or the hypothalamus. HH is associated with obesity; it has also been observed to be more prevalent in nondiabetic MetSyn subjects. Indeed, young patients with type 2 diabetes, but not type 1 diabetes, have an increased prevalence of HH, and in young men aged 20 to 39 years who have no manifestations of MetSyn a low testosterone level predicts the development of MetSyn features in later years.

The reason for the increased prevalence of HH with MetSyn is that both of these conditions are associated with increased peritoneal fat. Peritoneal fat, compared with subcutaneous fat, has an increased activity of the enzyme aromatase, which converts androgens and androgen precursors to estrogen. Elevated estrogen levels at the level of the hypothalamus suppress the production and release of gonadotrophin releasing hormone (GRH), which, in turn, results in decreased release of the gonadotrophins FSH and LH. Decreased LH production results in decreased testosterone production from the testicles and low serum testosterone levels. Lower testosterone levels result in decreased libido, anemia, osteoporosis, lower prostate specific antigen (PSA) levels, decreased muscle strength, asthenia, and fatigue. Testosterone deficiency also causes insulin resistance or worsens existing insulin resistance, leading to an increased risk of advancement to diabetes in the glucose-intolerant or insulin-resistant subject or worsening of glycemic control in the established diabetic patient.

Testosterone deficiency also results in decreased activity of the beta-adrenergic receptors, which are situated on the surface of the adipocytes. This leads to increased lipoprotein lipase activity, which, in turn, increases the release of FFAs from the abdominal, but not subcutaneous, adipocytes and worsening of MetSyn. In addition, the loss of adipocyte beta-adrenergic activity decreases energy utilization and causes weight gain. In animals, diminished beta-adrenergic responsiveness is induced by castration and reversed with testosterone replacement therapy. In addition, replacement of testosterone has the effect of redistributing the fat mass from the peritoneal cavity to the periphery, which will improve the manifestations of MetSyn.

NEPHROLITHIASIS

The incidence of nephrolithiasis is increased with both obesity and diabetes, and an increased excretion of calcium has been shown in both of these conditions. However, hypercalciuria is not related to MetSyn, and in the diabetic patient tends to resolve with improved glycemic control. MetSyn, although not associated with hypercalciuria, does predispose one to the development of calcium-containing stones by lowering the production and excretion of urinary citrate. In a study of nondiabetic calcium stone formers, those with the highest levels of insulin resistance had the lowest excretion of citrate. This prospective study is in keeping with epidemiological studies that have shown an association among kidney stones, obesity, hypertension, and diabetes.

Unlike hypercalciuria, uricosuria is clearly associated with MetSyn and is accompanied by an increase in nephrolithiasis. Hyperuricemia, a common feature of MetSyn, contributes to the formation of uric acid stones, as do the high insulin levels that are typically present in individuals with MetSyn. Hyperinsulinemia causes acidic urine by augmenting acid production and decreasing the production of ammonia, so that less acid is excreted as ammonia. Pure uric acid stone formers have a higher incidence of diabetes, impaired glucose tolerance, insulin resistance, and MetSyn.

BENIGN PROSTATIC HYPERTROPHY

Benign prostatic hypertrophy (BPH) has been shown to be associated with obesity, especially abdominal obesity, and higher insulin levels. Men with rapidly enlarging prostates have been shown to have a higher prevalence of diabetes, hypertension, abdominal obesity, lower HDL cholesterol levels, and higher fasting insulin levels. Prostatic growth as assessed by ultrasound is positively correlated with obesity, diastolic blood pressure, and fasting insulin levels and negatively with HDL cholesterol levels.

Prostatic growth is also associated not only with low testosterone and higher estradiol levels, but also with high insulin levels, owing to the ability of insulin to function as a growth factor. Therefore, because all three of these risk factors for prostatic growth—low testosterone, high estradiol, and high insulin—are associated with MetSyn, the link between prostate enlargement and MetSyn is probably largely explained by increases in these three growth factors.

Symptoms related to BPH are also associated with MetSyn, but the increased frequency of these symptoms does not correlate with an increased prostatic mass. The likely reason for the increased symptom frequency with MetSyn is increased activity of the sympathetic nervous system. Another reason is that the inflammation and oxidative stress associated with MetSyn can precipitate symptoms in a previously asymptomatic individual with an enlarged prostate.

CHRONIC KIDNEY DISEASE

MetSyn is undoubtedly associated with chronic kidney disease (CKD) and end-stage renal disease (ESRD). The association of MetSyn with risk factors such as diabetes, hypertension, albuminuria, oxidative stress, and endothelial dysfunction are also associated with CKD and ESRD and thus preclude MetSyn from being validated as an independent risk factor. However, studies comparing hypertensive patients with or without the features of MetSyn have shown that even with equivalent control of hypertension the deterioration in renal function is accelerated in the presence of MetSyn features. Additionally, the presence of MetSyn has been shown to be an independent risk factor for an accelerated decline in renal function.

In animal models of diabetic nephropathy, the expression of PPAR gamma receptor on the glomerular podocytes is increased. In an animal model of diabetic nephropathy where insulin injections were compared with utilization of pioglitazone while maintaining similar HbA1c levels, only pioglitazone inhibited glomerular hypertrophy and mesangial matrix expansion and reduced glucose-induced G_1-phase cell cycle arrest. A study utilizing rosiglitazone in diabetic nephropathy found that rosiglitazone slowed the decline in renal function.

Other possible reasons for the association of MetSyn and kidney disease are that hyperinsulinemia causes preglomerular vasodilatation and postglomerular vasoconstriction

The resultant increase in intraglomerular pressure leads to hyperfiltration, glomerulomegaly, and eventually glomerulosclerosis. Efferent arteriolar constriction and afferent arteriolar dilatation stimulate activity of the RAAS, and afferent arteriolar dilation also increases sodium absorption. Hyperinsulinemia increases glomerular permeability by stimulating mesangial cells to synthesize matrix glycoprotein, which contributes to the development of glomerulosclerosis. In addition, lipotoxicity associated with MetSyn in the proximal tubular cells leads to inflammation, apoptosis, and fibrosis. Fibrosis is also directly stimulated by the inflammation and endothelial dysfunction associated with MetSyn.

CONCLUSION

Manifestations of MetSyn in the genitourinary tract include PCOS, premature pubarche, and postmenopausal hyperandrogenemia in the female. In the male, MetSyn is associated with hypothalamic hypogonadism and BPH. MetSyn is also associated with an increased incidence of both calcium oxalate and uric acid stones and accelerates the progression of CKD.

Chapter 9

Central Nervous System Manifestations of the Metabolic Syndrome

METABOLIC SYNDROME AND CEREBROVASCULAR DISEASE

The two major risk factors for stroke—diabetes and hypertension—are both manifestations of the MetSyn. Although other manifestations of the MetSyn add to the stoke risk, the presence of MetSyn itself has been shown to be an independent stroke risk factor.

The incidence of hemorrhagic stroke is not increased with MetSyn. However, the incidence of nonhemorrhagic stroke (atherosclerotic extracranial and intracranial stroke, embolic and lacunar infarcts) is increased in MetSyn. Lacunar infarcts, which are due to fibrinoid necrosis in the microvascular circulation, causing subcortical and sometimes silent infarcts, are associated with diabetes and/or hypertension, and thus are also commonly associated with MetSyn. However, MetSyn also increases the risk of embolic and athero sclerotic stroke.

An increase in carotid intima-medial thickening is independently associated with MetSyn. Extracranial large artery atherosclerosis in whites has been associated with MetSyn; in other races there is an association with intracranial large vessel atherosclerosis. Nevertheless, embolic strokes from extracranial sites account for the majority of the increased incidence of stroke with MetSyn, and embolic strokes, particularly following revascularization of the coronary and carotid arteries, have been associated with MetSyn. In addition, because atrial fibrillation is more common in MetSyn, the left atrium is a common source of emboli.

DEMENTIA AND METABOLIC SYNDROME

In multiple studies, MetSyn has been shown to be a risk factor for accelerated cognitive ageing. Based on the association of MetSyn with cerebrovascular disease, the increased association of MetSyn with dementia could be concluded to be due to an increased prevalence of vascular or multi-infarct dementia. However, although there is an increase in vascular dementia with MetSyn, the major reason for the increased prevalence of accelerated cognitive ageing with MetSyn is Alzheimer's disease (AD).

ALZHEIMER'S DISEASE AND METABOLIC SYNDROME

Alzheimer's disease is associated with accumulation of amyloid plaque, especially in the temporal, frontal, and parietal lobes, leading to neurodegenerative disease and impaired memory. In the areas of the brain where amyloid plaque accumulates, positron emission tomography (PET) scans show decreased uptake of glucose in patients with MetSyn. It has been proposed that AD is associated not only with MetSyn, but also with a specific cerebro-cortical insulin resistance. It has been shown that during cerebral stimulation with insulin there is enhanced information processing in lean individuals, resulting in increases in both the beta and theta bands of spontaneous cortical activity. However, during cerebral stimulation in the obese, insulin does not increase beta activity and decreases theta activity, indicating that there is a specific cerebral insulin resistance in the obese. Carriers of the ARG allele, which is associated with genetic insulin resistance, show a more intense insulin-resistance pattern with decreased beta and no theta activity on cerebral stimulation with insulin. Therefore, with both genetic and acquired MetSyn there is an association with cerebrocortical insulin resistance, which may be due to defective transport of glucose across the blood–brain barrier and/or an intraneuronal defect in insulin signaling.

Cerebrocortical insulin resistance might result in higher cerebral insulin levels and trigger the accumulation of beta-amyloid, which eventually coalesces to form the amyloid plaques that are the hallmark of AD.

A viable hypothesis for the accumulation of beta-amyloid is that the same degrading enzyme systems break down and clear both insulin and beta-amyloid. The preferred sub-strate for this enzyme is insulin, so that with cerebrocortical insulin resistance and cerebral hyperinsulinemia excess beta-amyloid accumulates and aggregates to form amyloid plaques. Increased cerebral beta-amyloid, in addition to impairing memory, increases the risk of neu-odegenerative disease.

Another hypothesis is that insulin increases the intracellular clearance of beta-amyloid and protects neurons from the toxic effects of amyloid, so that when insulin resistance devel-ops the neurons are unprotected.

An alternate theory is that instead of insulin resistance causing accumulation of beta-amyloid, it is the accumulation of beta-amyloid that causes cerebrocortical insulin resistance. Accumulation of beta amyloid has been shown to cause cerebrocortical insulin resistance that develops because of oligomers of amyloid-removing insulin receptors from the dendritic plasma membranes of neurons, especially in the hippocampus. With this theory, administering TZDs or insulin would protect against the removal of insulin receptors.

A vascular hypothesis for the association of cerebrocortical disease with insulin resistance has also been proposed. Insulin resistance causes downregulation of the phosphoinositide-3-kinase pathway. This pathway controls vasodilatation and upregulation of the mitogen-activation protein kinase pathway, which causes vasoconstriction. At autopsy, the brains of diabetic subjects with dementia have a higher concentration of microvascular lesions when compared with diabetic patients without dementia. Although these lesions were not the major reason for the cognitive defect noted among these patients, their presence points to a broad-based vascular dysfunction and another contributing factor in the cerebral dysfunction commonly seen in the diabetic individual.

Therefore, the treatment of MetSyn and insulin resistance theoretically might improve both memory and the pace of age-related cognitive decline.

THERAPY OF METABOLIC SYNDROME AND MANIFESTATIONS OF ALZHEIMER'S DEMENTIA

A prospective study in which AD patients were randomized to either placebo, nateglinide, or the TZD pioglitazone for 4 months showed increased glucose uptake in the classical AD areas in the pioglitazone-treated group but not in the nateglinide or placebo groups. Cognitive testing at 2 and 4 months in these subjects showed improvements in cognitive function in the TZD group, which paralleled the increased uptake of glucose in the AD areas.

PET scan studies have also shown that defects in word memory testing closely matched decreased glucose uptake in the frontal cortex. Glucose uptake was impaired more in those with impaired glucose tolerance and even more in those with type 2 diabetes.

To increase cerebral insulin levels, which may overcome cerebral insulin resistance, the use of nasal insulin, which features a more direct route to the brain, has been shown to improve memory by as much as 50% even in healthy adults. In a study of 22 healthy adults and 46 older subjects with memory impairment, nasal insulin was compared with saline and no nasal infusion. Both the healthy adults and older adults with memory problems showed an improvement in memory within 15 minutes, and the improvement in memory was much greater in the older memory-impaired subjects.

Therefore, MetSyn therapies designed to overcome cerebrocortical insulin resistance through use of TZDs or intranasal insulin improve cognitive function.

PERIPHERAL NEUROPATHY AND METABOLIC SYNDROME

In the type 2 diabetic subject, symptomatic neuropathy is often present at the time of diagnosis. Although the presence of neuropathy at diagnosis could be associated with a delayed diagnosis of diabetes and prolonged hyperglycemia, the likely cause of the neuropathy in these patients is the presence of MetSyn predating the development of diabetes.

A study of 548 subjects with type 2 diabetes showed that those with more than three features of MetSyn were twice as likely to have neuropathy. Long-term follow up of 2,000 type 1 diabetic subjects who at baseline had no manifestations of neuropathy showed that the presence of features of MetSyn were predictive for developing neuropathy.

Idiopathic neuropathy, a condition that by definition occurs in an individual without diabetes or glucose intolerance, is also associated with MetSyn. A study of 219 subjects with idiopathic neuropathy showed a higher prevalence of the features of MetSyn compared with healthy controls. Additionally, when subjects with idiopathic neuropathy were compared with diabetic subjects who did not have neuropathy, there was a higher prevalence of hyperlipidemia (low HDL and increased triglycerides). Indeed, the presence of hypertriglyceridemia itself has been shown to be independently associated with neuropathy. In the Fenofibrate Intervention and Event Lowering in Diabetes (FIELD) study, fenofibrate, which reduces triglyceride levels, was associated with a decrease in amputations that were most likely to be due to decreased development of neuropathy.

Why is neuropathy associated with MetSyn? The likely pathophysiological reason is endothelial dysfunction. Especially in type 2 diabetic patients with distal symmetrical polyneuropathy, nerve biopsies show asymmetrical demyelination associated with occlusions of the vasa nervorum. Thus, the association of MetSyn with neuropathy is most likely vascular and due to endothelial dysfunction affecting the microvasculature.

CONCLUSIONS

MetSyn is associated with an increased incidence of nonhemorrhagic stroke, silent cerebral infarct, and multi-infarct dementia. Cerebrocortical insulin resistance and higher insulin levels are associated with MetSyn. Increased cerebrocortical insulin levels, probably by overwhelming the degrading enzymes that are common to both insulin and beta-amyloid, decreases the breakdown of beta-amyloid, leading to its coalescence into amyloid plaque. These plaques can then accumulate in the areas of the brain associated with AD. Overcoming or reducing the cerebrocortical insulin resistance results in increased cerebral glucose uptake on PET scans of the brains of AD patients and improved memory and cognition. Peripheral neuropathy due to endothelial dysfunction is associated with MetSyn even in the absence of diabetes or glucose intolerance.

Chapter 10

Respiratory Manifestation of Metabolic Syndrome

LUNG FUNCTION AND METABOLIC SYNDROME

Impaired lung function is a novel risk factor for insulin resistance, glucose intolerance, and type 2 diabetes. A 20-year prospective study found that subjects with decreased vital capacity, forced expiratory volume in 1 second (FEV_1), and lower mid-expiratory flow rate were more likely to develop insulin resistance and hyperinsulinemia, even when corrections were made for age, smoking, and obesity. Hypoxia, probably by inducing oxidative stress and endothelial dysfunction, is also associated with MetSyn; even short-term exposure to hypoxia decreases insulin sensitivity.

A possible explanation for the association of MetSyn and lung function is that decreased lung volumes are associated with low birth weight, and low birth weight is also associated with MetSyn. Another possibility is that inflammatory proteins produced in the presence of chronic lung disease and alveolar damage, by escaping into the systemic circulation through a damaged alveolar–capillary barrier, precipitate the development of MetSyn.

Insulin receptors have been identified on type II pneumocytes, and in vitro studies have shown that the addition of insulin increases the production of surfactant from these cells. The presence of MetSyn and resistance to the action of insulin on the pneumocytes could lead to decreased surfactant production, with subsequent damage to the alveolocapillary membrane. Increased alveolar permeability could lead to deposition of protein and lipid within the lung, leading to decreased compliance.

EXERCISE CAPACITY AND METABOLIC SYNDROME

The presence of MetSyn has been consistently associated with decreased exercise capacity. This is most likely related to endothelial dysfunction, because administration of l-arginine, a precursor of nitric oxide, improves exercise capacity, as does the TZD rosiglitazone. Although rosiglitazone improves both oxidative stress and endothelial function, this may not be the only mechanism by which it improves exercise capacity, because MetSyn is associated with mitochondrial dysfunction and mitochondrial dysfunction is associated with defective exercise capacity. Therefore, improved mitochondrial function with the TZD rosiglitazone could explain the improvement in exercise tolerance that has been shown to occur with this class of drugs in type 2 diabetic subjects.

SLEEP APNEA SYNDROME AND METABOLIC SYNDROME

Sleep apnea syndrome (SAS) is not localized to the respiratory tract but is a systemic disease that is typically associated with MetSyn. Independent of obesity, sleep apnea has been associated with increased visceral fat, hyperinsulinemia, and increased TNF-α and IL6 levels. Elevations in TNF-α and IL6 are at least partially responsible for the daytime sleepiness associated with SAS. Women with PCOS are more likely to have sleep disorder breathing and daytime sleepiness. Postmenopausal women also have an increased prevalence of SAS, which can be reduced significantly with hormone replacement therapy, improving the manifestations of MetSyn (see Chapter 13). Therapy of SAS with continuous positive airway pressure (CPAP) decreases visceral fat, cytokine levels, and insulin resistance. TNF-α antagonists, exercise, and weight loss also improve the manifestation of SAS.

SAS is also associated with defective central neural mechanisms, such as decreased secretion of corticotrophin releasing hormone (CRH) from the hypothalamus, resulting in decreased adrenocorticotropic hormone (ACTH) production by the anterior pituitary gland and low cortisol levels. In addition to inflammation and neurohormonal activation, SAS is also associated with sympathetic activation. As a result, patients with SAS, like those with MetSyn, are "nondippers" due to increased sympathetic activation and the loss of a physiological decrease in catecholamines during sleep, which results in an increased incidence of acute CV events in the early morning hours.

Obstructive breathing causes fragmentation of sleep and hypoxia, both of which stimulate inflammation and neurohormonal and sympathetic activation, all of which lead to manifestations of MetSyn. The truncal and neck obesity (neck circumference greater than 17 inches (43 cm) in a man and 13 inches (33 cm) in a woman) that is a fundamental cause of MetSyn is also causal in the genesis of SAS. Thus, MetSyn and SAS are interrelated and inseparable, with MetSyn leading to SAS and SAS leading to MetSyn.

SLEEP DEPRIVATION AND METABOLIC SYNDROME

Sleep deprivation, like SAS, increases insulin resistance. A crossover study of normal volunteers showed increased insulin resistance when sleep was restricted to 5.5 hours compared with when 8.5 hours of sleep were allowed. Sleep deprivation caused a 25% increase in nocturnal catecholamine levels, a delayed drop in cortisol after the onset of sleep, and weight gain, which intensified insulin resistance and other MetSyn features. Sleep deprivation is also associated with increased incidence of diabetes, cardiac events, and mortality.

A possible explanation for these associations is that the same genes that regulate insulin signaling also regulate the body's "sleep–wake cycle." Mice with genetic dysfunctional diurnal variation become obese and develop diabetes. Therefore, our internal clocks may be reset by dysfunction of the insulin-signaling system.

CONCLUSION

MetSyn is associated with decreased exercise capacity, SAS, and sleep deprivation. Interventions to improve the manifestations of MetSyn improve lung function and sleep quality, and therapy of SAS and sleep deprivation improve the manifestations of MetSyn.

Chapter 11

Cancer and the Metabolic Syndrome

ASSOCIATION OF METABOLIC SYNDROME WITH CANCER

The components of MetSyn have been individually linked with the development of cancer. In the Chicago Heart Association Detection Project in Industry study, after the exclusion of diabetes, the relative risk of colorectal-related cancer mortality was increased significantly in men (67%) and nonsignificantly in women (29%) with features of MetSyn. Similarly, in the Risk Factors and Life Expectancy studies, death from colorectal cancer was increased threefold in women, but not in men. The features of MetSyn and the effect of individual components of MetSyn were additive.

Obesity, whether expressed as BMI or as waist-to-hip ratio, is associated with increased incidences of cancers of the colon, breast (postmenopausal), endometrium, esophagus, liver, gallbladder, stomach, pancreas, and kidney. In addition, obesity is associated with increased cancer mortality and contributes to in excess of 100,000 cancer deaths per year in the United States. Adult weight gain is associated with an increased risk of both postmenopausal breast cancer and endometrial cancer; conversely, weight loss significantly decreases the risk of cancer in premenopausal, but not postmenopausal, females.

Exercise has been shown to decrease the risk of developing cancer. Forty-eight studies of colorectal cancer found that exercise resulted in a "dose-related" reduction in the risk of developing a malignant colonic neoplasm. Similarly, in 26 of 41 studies of breast cancer exercise decreased the risk—again, in a "dose-related" way—of both peri- and postmenopausal breast cancer.

An elevated fasting glucose level is also associated with an increased risk of cancer, particularly cancers of the pancreas, liver, and kidney, and an increase in mortality with multiple cancers. The presence of diabetes is also associated with increased incidences of and mortality from pancreatic, hepatic, endometrial, cervical, and breast cancers.

In nondiabetic subjects, fasting insulin levels are significantly and independently associated with the development of colorectal, breast, endometrial, and prostate cancers. Diabetic subjects who use insulin or sulfonylureas, which increase insulin levels, have a higher risk of developing cancer. In contrast, diabetic subjects on metformin, which lowers insulin levels, have a lower risk of developing cancer. In the Tayside study of patients with new-onset type 2 diabetes, the risk of cancer was 11.6% in those treated with insulin therapy and 7.3% in those treated with metformin. The median time to develop a cancer was 2.6 years with insulin therapy and 3.5 years with metformin therapy, with the hazard ratio for cancer being 0.46 with metformin when compared with insulin. Another population study showed a cancer mortality rate of 3.5% with metformin, 4.9% with sulfonylureas, and 5.8% with insulin use. In this study, after multivariate analysis, compared with metformin users, users of sulfonylureas had a 30% increase and users of insulin a 90% increase in cancer-related mortality.

Having a MetSyn lipid pattern of low HDL and elevated triglyceride levels is a risk factor for cancers of the colon, breast, and prostate. Another component of MetSyn, systolic hypertension, has been associated with a 23% increase in cancer-related morality, a 75% increase in renal cancer death, and an increase in the prevalence of endometrial cancer.

Therefore, the frequency of cancers and cancer-related mortality increases with both MetSyn and its various components. An independent association with MetSyn has been shown with cancers of the pancreas, liver, biliary tract, colorectal (in men only), breast, endometrium, and urinary tract. Why are these cancers associated with MetSyn?

ETIOLOGY OF INCREASED CANCER RISK AND MORTALITY WITH METABOLIC SYNDROME

The major factor in the increased cancer risk and mortality that occurs with MetSyn would seem to be hyperinsulinemia. Insulin is an anabolic hormone that can directly stimulate cell proliferation. Insulin's effect may also be indirect in that it increases the number of hepatic receptors for growth hormone so that the hepatic production of IGF_1 is increased. Insulin can also increase the availability IGF_1 to the tissues by decreasing the hepatic production of its carrier protein (IGFBP) so that more unbound IGF_1 is available to stimulate IGF_1 receptors on both normal and cancer cells. IGF_1 causes cell proliferation as well as increasing the blood and nutrient supply to these cells through increased angiogenesis. Increased angiogenesis caused by increased IGF_1 receptor activity also facilitates metastatic spread and has an anti-apoptotic effect, which further increases tumor growth. Therefore, by increasing proliferation and angiogenesis and decreasing apoptosis, increased IGF_1 levels induced by hyperinsulinemia increase tumor growth and spread.

Tumor cell growth, particularly with breast and endometrial cancers, is facilitated by elevated estrogen levels caused by excessive activity of the aromatase enzyme, which facilitates the production of estrogens from its androgenic precursors. The activity of aromatase has been shown to be increased in the presence of excessive peritoneal fat. Excessive intra-abdominal fat also produces excessive TNF-α and IL6, which, in conjunction with augmented levels of prostaglandins produced by fibroblasts, increase aromatase activity.

Increased leptin levels, which are typical of obesity and MetSyn, have been associated with prostate, colon, breast, and endometrial cancers. In vitro, the addition of leptin to a cell culture promotes the growth of leukemia cells. Leptin, by increasing the production of metallo-proteinases and by promoting angiogenesis, is associated with increased metastatic activity.

Adiponectin, which is typically decreased in MetSyn, has been associated with decreased development of cancers of the breast, endometrium, and stomach. Adiponectin's primary action is activation of 5-AMPK in multiple tissues. Interestingly, metformin has an effect on the same enzyme system, which may at least partially explain why metformin protects the diabetic patient from developing the cancers that are increased in individuals with MetSyn and diabetes. Increased activity of 5-AMPK, which increases energy levels within the cell (see Chapter 4), is thought to inhibit both tumor formation and tumor growth.

Vascular endothelial growth factor (VEGF) is secreted by adipocytes, particularly peritoneal adipocytes, and its production is stimulated by hypoxia, insulin, IGF-1, estrogen, TNF-α, and leptin. VEGF, the levels of which are increased in MetSyn, has been shown to play a major role in angiogenesis, tumor progression, and metastatic activity.

Inflammation, which is also associated with MetSyn, leads to oxidative stress, which promotes the development and progression of tumors. Chronic low-grade inflammation is a risk factor for gastric, pancreatic, hepatic, esophageal, bladder, and colorectal cancers. Inflammation has been shown to both increase the growth of tumor cells and suppress apoptosis. Oxidative stress, which is associated with inflammation, damages DNA and up-regulates cyclooxygenase-2 (COX-2) by multiple pathways. Inflammation and oxidative stress are associated with cancers of breast, colon, and prostate.

Cancer cells, owing to their increased metabolic rate, have increased glucose requirements. Cancer cells increase the activity of glucose transporters, particularly GLUT-1, to adapt to this increased need. Thus energy restriction, at least in primate studies, inhibits the development and progression of tumors. In glucose-intolerant or diabetic subjects, an increased availability of glucose could explain the increased risk of developing certain, but not all, cancer types, and could also explain the increased mortality associated with these and other cancers in the diabetic subject.

COMBATING INCREASED CANCER INCIDENCE AND MORTALITY IN METABOLIC SYNDROME

Intuitively, maintaining a body weight as close to normal as possible should protect against the development of the cancers associated with MetSyn. To combat the inflammation and oxidative stress associated with MetSyn, a diet rich in antioxidants, such as those found in vegetables and fruits (especially deeply pigmented, less-processed varieties), olive oil, tea, soy, red wine, and nuts (especially pecans and pistachios), should be followed. A diet that is high in nutrients and low in calorie density has been shown to protect against the development of both breast and colon cancer. The American Institute of Cancer Research has stated that weight maintenance, daily exercise, breastfeeding of babies, and limiting alcohol intake could result in as much as a 50% reduction in the incidence of breast cancer.

Controlling any elevation of glucose is important not only to avoid oxidative stress but also to "starve" cancer cells that need glucose to grow. The method by which glucose levels are lowered is also important. Metformin protects against the development and progression of cancers by lowering insulin levels and stimulating 5-AMPK. However, inducing hyperinsulinemia, either through injection of insulin or stimulation of insulin secretion and release from the pancreas with a sulfonylurea or the meglitinides, increases tumor growth through increased proliferation, angiogenesis, and suppression of apoptosis. Also, increased angiogenesis not only enables tumor growth but also promotes metastatic activity and increases mortality.

The type of insulin utilized may also be important. Compared with recombinant–DNA-derived human insulin, short-acting insulin analogues, even when combined with protamine, have not been shown to further increase the risk of developing the cancers that are associated with insulin use. However, the long-acting insulin analog glargine may be associated with an increased incidence of cancers of the pancreas, breast, and prostate. Although the data on glargine are conflicting, if confirmed to be true, it could be due to an increased mitogenic effect of this insulin caused by a prolonged attachment to the insulin receptor and cross-reactivity with the IGF_1 receptor.

CONCLUSION

MetSyn and/or its individual components are associated with an increased risk of cancers of the pancreas, biliary tract, liver, stomach, colon, rectum, breast, endometrium, and urinary tract. In addition, MetSyn and/or its components are associated with an increased risk of mortality from multiple cancers. The likely causative factors are increased activity of insulin, IGF_1, aromatases, adipocytokines (TNF-α and leptin), and VEGF and decreased adiponectin activity. The chronically elevated levels of inflammation and oxidative stress, as well as increased availability of glucose to tumors, are additional factors magnifying cancer risk in MetSyn individuals. Antioxidant intake, control of glucose, normalization of body weight, and the use of metformin in MetSyn and diabetic subjects will help protect against the development and spread of cancer. Whenever possible, the use of sulfonylureas, meglitinides, and insulin should be avoided in the diabetic patient. If insulin needs to be utilized, pending the availability of more definitive information, the long-acting insulin analog glargine should be used with caution.

Chapter 12

Factors that Worsen Metabolic Syndrome

GENETICS AND THE INTRAUTERINE ENVIRONMENT

Fifty percent of MetSyn is due to genetics and/or the uterine environment. During critical periods of intrauterine development, to survive and conserve energy the fetus becomes resistant to the action of insulin. Although later in life this in–utero-acquired insulin resistance may help protect against starvation, in the modern day environment of excessive availability and utilization of calories, fats, and carbohydrates this resistance to the action of insulin is pathological. This is particularly true if following the birth of a small baby "catch-up" growth occurs. The finding that the intrauterine environment, through "genetic imprinting," is more important than the true genetics of the fetus comes from the recent observation that children born to mothers who have previously lost weight through bariatric surgery are less resistant to the action of insulin than are those born at the time of the previous greater maternal obesity.

LOW BIRTH WEIGHT

Birth weight is a major predictor for development of MetSyn. Small women [BMI less than 18 and/or height less than 60 inches (152 cm)] and small animals are protected from having a large first baby due to both the limited uterine environment and the effect of suppressing of paternal genes through decreased expression of growth factors and growth factor receptors. The offspring of small women, even though of small stature, have increased subscapular fat, and the volume of this fat has been shown to be proportional to the volume of peritoneal fat. Therefore, these babies already have a neonatal form of MetSyn at birth, and indeed when reassessed at age 8 already have most of the characteristics of MetSyn. Increased levels of insulin in the umbilical cord blood of small babies is further evidence that some elements of MetSyn are present at birth. Therefore, genetics, the uterine environment, and the amount of postnatal growth interact to set the stage for MetSyn at birth and predispose the individual to the overt manifestation of this malady later in life.

In Hertfordshire, England, 64-year-old men who were small at birth were more likely to have diabetes or impaired glucose tolerance. In Danish identical twins, if only one of the twins had diabetes the diabetic twin was found to weigh less at birth than the nondiabetic twin. In Holland during World War II, rationing of food resulted in a lower birth weight and an increased frequency of diabetes later in life. These and more than 40 other epidemiological studies have confirmed the association of low birth weight with mitochondrial dysfunction, MetSyn, diabetes, hypertension, and breast cancer.

Compared with well-fed pregnant rats, pregnant rats fed a low-protein (8% versus 20%) isocaloric diet during pregnancy and lactation had smaller offspring that had a higher incidence of MetSyn, beta cell dysfunction, and dysglycemia. Furthermore, the pancreatic islet cells were smaller and hypovascular and had lower insulin content. The release of insulin was less responsive to stimulation with either glucose or amino acids in these animals.

Thus the concept of the development of a "thrifty phenotype" in response to gestational malnutrition due either to starvation or placental dysfunction has been proposed. The concept is that by protecting the brain at the expense of other organs (including the pancreas) to facilitate postnatal survival the fetus enhances its ability to store fat, which leads to obesity, insulin resistance, and type 2 diabetes.

ENVIRONMENTAL FACTORS

MetSyn is worsened by ageing, loss of muscle mass, obesity, and a sedentary lifestyle. The development of anxiety, by increasing catecholamine levels, will worsen MetSyn. Depression, not only by increasing catecholamine levels, but also by increasing glucocorticoid production with a loss of diurnal variation, worsens MetSyn. Thus, a depressed diabetic patient may need a major increase in insulin dosage following the development of depression and a major decrease in the insulin dose when depression is alleviated. Indeed, in many cases the only way to obtain glycemic control in the depressed diabetic patient is to administer antidepressants.

Infection, by increasing cytokine production, catecholamines, and cortisol, will also worsen MetSyn. Sometimes the infection may be chronic, asymptomatic, and not clinically obvious. For example, in a diabetic patient hyperglycemia may result from a tooth abscess or a silent urinary tract infection. A course of antibiotics and/or drainage of an abscess will rapidly improve the glycemic control.

Acute severe illnesses also worsen MetSyn. Clinically silent (asymptomatic) myocardial infarctions commonly occur in the diabetic patient. These patients may present with an acute increase in glucose and ketone levels due to the acute worsening of MetSyn caused by the MI. Acutely, a MI is often accompanied by a significant decrease in HDL cholesterol and an increase in triglyceride levels. Similarly, the development of a malignancy can result in similar changes in lipid and glucose levels due to the excessive cytokines produced by the tumor, which worsen the manifestations of MetSyn.

DIETARY FACTORS

In Ireland in 1839 the diet of a typical farm worker was one of potatoes and skim milk, and for all practical purposes diabetes seldom, if ever, occurred. Following the "potato famine," sugar, starch, fat, and eggs were introduced into the Irish diet, which resulted in a sharp increase in the intake of calories and incidence of death due to diabetes. Interestingly, the only two times that the incidence of diabetes-related death decreased was following the World Wars when there was rationing of food.

In the United States, over the past 50 years very significant changes in nutrition and exercise have occurred. Food preparation has moved from the family kitchen to commercial purveyors and processors of calorie-dense, lipid-rich foods. Over this 50-year period, there has

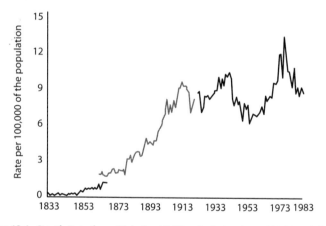

Figure 12.1. Death Rate from Diabetes Mellitus in Ireland per 100,000 of the Population 1833–1983

Source: Crawford EM. Death Rates from diabetes mellitus in Ireland, 1833–1983: a historical commentary. *Ulster Medical Journal.* 1987;56(2):109–115. Reprinted by permission of the Ulster Medical Society.

been an average daily increase in calorie intake of 168 calories in men and 355 calories in women. Physical activities that 50 years ago were associated with normal life have been substantially decreased or eliminated. Because of these changes in diet and activity, two-thirds of Americans are overweight or obese. Utilization of "fast-food" restaurants where a 630-calorie

Table 12.1. Weekly Food Rations of Irish Laborers (Co. Tipperary) 1839 and 1863

1839	1863
(per laboring man)	(for a 7-person family)
63–94 1/2 lb. potatoes	7 lb. flour
21–42 pt. skim milk	56 lb. Indian meal
	140 lb. potatoes
	1-1/2 lb. sugar
	2 lb. butter
	2 lb. meat
	56 pt. skim milk
	14 eggs

Source: Sixth annual report of the Poor Law Commissioners, BPP1840 (245) XVII, Appendix D: 244, Sixth report of the Medical Officer of the Privy Council, BPP 1864 (3416) XXVIII: 324.

chocolate chip muffin, a 1,300-calorie hamburger with cheese and fries, or a 1,610-calorie meal of three pieces of fried chicken with rice, coleslaw, and biscuit are readily available has worsened the situation.

Although the United States leads the world in obesity, with 34% of the population having a BMI of over 30, the United Kingdom is a close second, with 24% being obese, and European countries are in the intermediate range, with obesity rates ranging from 11% to 14%. Asian countries, to date, have not followed the Western world, but with Westernization of the diet increases in the rates of obesity in Asian countries are inevitable.

Although an excessive calorie intake will result in obesity, which will worsen MetSyn, the components of the diet are also important, because MetSyn is more likely to be caused or worsened by a diet that is high in saturated fat and/or sugar. Fructose, which is a component of high-fructose corn syrup, and sucrose are the nutrients that are most detrimental. Due to the use of high-fructose corn syrup in manufactured foods, the intake of fructose has increased by 25% over the past 40 years. A high fructose intake, by decreasing the production of leptin and not suppressing the production of ghrelin, is associated with decreased satiety, increased calorie intake, decreased energy expenditure, weight gain, and acute and chronic increases in cortisol and insulin levels due to increased resistance to the action of insulin in the myocytes, adipocytes, and hepatocytes. Increased fructose intake also results in increased hepatic lipogenesis through increased activity of hepatic acetyl CoA, which leads to increased triglyceride and VLDL levels and elevated postprandial triglyceride (a major cardiac risk factor) (See Table 12.2).

Although weight loss is difficult in our modern environment, for most people who lose weight it is almost impossible to maintain the weight loss. This is because with weight loss the appetite-stimulating hormones (ghrelin, insulin, and cortisol) are elevated and the appetite-suppressing hormones (leptin, GLP$_1$, cholecystokinin, neuropeptide YY, and oxyntomodulin) are decreased in patients who have lost weight. Foods that increase the appetite-stimulating hormones, such as sweets, potatoes, juices, refined breakfast cereals, white bread, rice, and preprandial alcohol, should be avoided. Foods that suppress the appetite-stimulating

Table 12.2. Fructose (Corn Syrup) or Sucrose Versus Glucose

- No simulation of insulin secretion
- Decreased leptin
- Decreased suppression of ghrelin
- Decreased satiety
- Increased calorie intake
- Decreased energy expenditure
- Weight gain
- Acute and chronic increases in insulin resistance

Source: Swarbick MM. *Br J Natr.* (2008)1–6; Teff K. *J Clin Endocrinol Metab.* (2004)89:2963–72; Teff K. *Diabetes.* (2005)A385.

hormones and that stimulate the appetite-suppressing hormones—high-fiber vegetables and fruits and the proteins obtained from chicken and fish—should be utilized.

CIGARETTE SMOKING

Cigarette smoking worsens MetSyn. Physicians who smoke over 20 cigarettes per day have a 70% increased chance of developing type 2 diabetes. In the CARDIA study, smokers increased their chances of developing diabetes by 65%, and for every 10-year-pack history there was an 18% increase in the incidence of diabetes. Unfortunately, those exposed to secondhand smoke also increased their chances of developing diabetes by 35%.

HYPOGONADISM

That testosterone depletion worsens MetSyn was addressed in Chapter 8. Interestingly, androgen-deprivation therapy prescribed to cure or ameliorate prostate cancer, while initially decreasing mortality after 6 months and while still improving survival from prostate cancer, has no further effect on total mortality. This is because the improvement in deaths related to prostate cancer is negated by an increase in CV death, which is largely due to worsening of the manifestations of MetSyn through androgen deprivation.

Androgen-deprivation therapy that utilizes gonadotrophin antagonists has also been shown to significantly increase the incidence of diabetes by 44%, CAD by 16%, MI by 11%, and sudden cardiac death by 16%. Therefore, due to worsening of MetSyn, the risk-to-benefit ratio of androgen-deprivation therapy for prostate cancer needs to be closely evaluated in an ongoing fashion.

Hypoestrogenemic females have very high FFA levels, and because of this the post-menopausal state is associated with MetSyn. An example of worsening of MetSyn with estrogen deficiency is that hypertension commonly develops soon after the menopause. Postmenopausal utilization of estrogen replacement therapy, by reducing insulin resistance, is associated with a 30% decrease in the development of diabetes. Unfortunately, in the type 2 diabetic female the use of postmenopausal hormone replacement therapy results in a 3.2-fold increase in mortality, a 4.2-fold increase in the development of CAD, and a 9.2-fold greater incidence of MI.

The differences between diabetic and nondiabetic females in the CV effects of hormone replacement therapy can be explained by the presence of preexisting CAD. It has clearly been shown that the initiation of estrogen replacement therapy in women in whom CAD is not present (i.e., hormone replacement therapy is initiated at the time of menopause) decreases the incidence of cardiac mortality and cardiac events. Alternatively, with preexisting CAD, estrogen therapy increases cardiac events and mortality. Unfortunately, at the time of menopause, patients with diabetes and/or MetSyn probably have established CAD.

PHARMACOLOGICAL AGENTS THAT WORSEN METABOLIC SYNDROME

Thiazide diuretics used in doses equivalent to 50 mg hydrochlorothiazide (HCTZ) that were utilized in studies such as the Antihypertensive and Lipid Lowering Treatment to Prevent Heart Attack Triad (ALLHAT) study worsened MetSyn and increased the incidence of diabetes by 38%. However, lower doses, such as 12.5 mg daily HCTZ, do not significantly increase the risk of MetSyn or diabetes, as was shown in the Atherosclerosis Risk in the Community (ARIC) study. Diuretic-induced salt depletion stimulates both the RAAS and the sympathetic nervous system, increasing insulin resistance and the risk of developing MetSyn and type 2 diabetes. Therefore, monotherapy of essential hypertension with diuretics may cause or worsen MetSyn.

Nicotinic acid, when used in doses of greater than 1 gram per day, results in an initial decrease in FFA levels, followed a few hours later by a rebound increase in FFAs that worsens the manifestations of MetSyn. However, the effect of nicotinic acid on MetSyn may over time decrease, and the cardiac risk of worsening MetSyn with nicotinic acid is more than outbalanced by the decreases in triglycerides and LDL cholesterol and the increases in HDL cholesterol and both LDL and HDL particle size. However, the risk of developing or worsening established diabetes is increased.

Perhaps the greatest offenders in increasing insulin resistance are the first- and second-generation vasoconstricting beta blockers. In the ARIC study, use of these beta blockers increased new-onset diabetes by 28%. In the LIFE trial, atenolol, when compared with the angiotensin receptor blocker losartan, which does not increase or decrease insulin resistance, increased the incidence of new-onset diabetes by 24%. In the COMET trial, subjects with HF treated with the second-generation beta blocker metoprolol sustained a 22% increase in the incidence of diabetes when compared with subjects utilizing the third-generation vasodilating beta blocker carvedilol. In the Glycemic Effects in Diabetes Mellitus: Carvedilol-Metoprolol Compariss (GEMINI) study of diabetic hypertensive subjects, carvedilol decreased HbA1c, insulin resistance, microalbuminuria, total cholesterol, and non-HDL cholesterol when compared with the vasoconstricting second-generation beta blocker metoprolol.

Why should metoprolol, but not carvedilol, increase the incidence of diabetes and worsen glycemic control, hyperlipidemia, and the features of MetSyn? Metoprolol, like almost all other first- and second-generation beta blockers, causes vasoconstriction, which decreases the surface area available for insulin-induced glucose utilization. However, carvedilol, which through its alpha$_1$ blocking effect is a vasodilating beta blocker, increases the surface area for insulin-induced glucose utilization, thus improving the manifestations of MetSyn.

Glucocorticoids in excess of physiological replacement dose worsen the manifestations of MetSyn. The effects of systemic cortisol levels within the normal range may be amplified by increased tissue cortisol levels. which occur due to increased activity of the enzyme 11β-OHSD-1.

The antiretroviral drugs used in the therapy of human immunodeficiency virus (HIV) also worsen MetSyn. This is due to both the HIV infection itself as well as utilization of antiretroviral drugs, which cause lipodystrophy by shifting fat from the subcutaneous space to the peritoneal cavity and liver, worsening the manifestations of MetSyn. Induction and worsening of MetSyn has therefore become a serious side effect of antiretroviral therapy. Although the use of TZDs with congenital lipodystrophies will cause a shift of fat toward the subcutaneous space, and away from the peritoneal cavity and the liver, this has not been the case with antiretroviral viral therapy. The probable explanation for this difference is that expression of PPAR gamma receptors may be decreased in the adipocytes, which are formed with antiretroviral therapy and not in the adipocytes associated with the congenital lipodystrophies.

The use of second-generation antipsychotic drugs (atypical antipsychotics) is associated with weight gain, worsening of the manifestations of MetSyn, and the development of diabetes. Although these drugs have enhanced the quality of life of the psychiatric patient, by not being as frequently associated with the irreversible extrapyramidal side effects that occur with the first-generation antipsychotics (phenothiazines), this group of drugs has replaced extrapyramidal effects with MetSyn and increased cardiometabolic risk. Although traditional antipsychotics act mainly of the dopamine D_2 receptors, atypical antipsychotics act on both the serotonin 2A and dopamine D_2 receptors. However, the weight gain seen with atypical antipsychotics is largely mediated through an effect on the histamine H_1 receptor, and the drugs that show the greatest affinity for this receptor (clozapine and olanzapine) are associated with the greatest weight gain. Acute decreases in insulin secretion or a shift to an increased oxidation of FFAs or an acute increase in glucagon production may be responsible for the increased frequency of diabetic ketoacidosis that occurs with these drugs in spite of the preservation of pancreatic beta cells and the retained capacity to secrete endogenous insulin. Another factor in the increased incidence of diabetes with these drugs may be damage to the pancreatic beta cells from pancreatitis, the incidence of which is increased with atypical antipsychotics. In a Veteran's Administration study of new-onset diabetes with atypical antipsychotics, the incidence of diabetes over a 1-year period was compared with that of the first-generation antipsychotic phenothiazine haloperidol. With risperidone and quetiapine, the incidence of diabetes was not increased; olanzapine significantly increased the development of diabetes by 84%. With olanzapine the increase in development of diabetes was not correlated with weight gain.

CONCLUSION

The prevalence of MetSyn is increased by genetics, low birth weight, catch-up growth, aging, loss of muscle mass, obesity, a sedentary lifestyle, infection, and major illnesses. Components of the diet, particularly fats and fructose, play a major role in the development of MetSyn. Glucocorticoids, vasoconstricting beta blockers, high-dose thiazides, nicotinic acid, antiretrovirals, and atypical antipsychotics also play a role in the development of or the worsening of the manifestations of MetSyn.

Chapter 13

Factors that Improve the Manifestations of Metabolic Syndrome

ENVIRONMENTAL FACTORS: DIET, WEIGHT LOSS, AND EXERCISE

The most potent factor in improving the manifestations of MetSyn is exercise. For every five miles a person walks each week there is a 6% decreased risk of developing diabetes, with a greater decrease occurring in those who are at higher risk (i.e., those with a strong family history of diabetes and those who are obese). Walking briskly for as little as 2.5 hours per week is enough to have a positive effect on the manifestations of MetSyn.

Obesity will worsen the manifestations of MetSyn, but a decrease in body weight of as little as 5% to 10%, which preferentially decreases peritoneal and hepatic fat, disproportionately improves the manifestations of MetSyn. Lifestyle intervention in the Diabetes Prevention Trial, which included a 7% weight loss, decreased the progression from impaired glucose tolerance to diabetes by 58%. Obese subjects who utilized adjustable gastric banding reduced their body weight by 24.6% and reduced insulin resistance by 34.5%. Subjects treating their obesity surgically with a Roux-en-Y gastric bypass reduced their body weight by 44% and their insulin resistance by 68.2%. Therefore, the greater the decrease in body weight, the greater the improvements in the manifestations of MetSyn.

DIETARY STRATEGIES

Daily calorie intake has increased approximately 250 calories over the past 30 years. Studies indicate that the epidemics of obesity, MetSyn, and type 2 diabetes can be largely accounted for by this increase in calorie intake.

Chronic intake of excess calories creates a vicious cycle whereby a diet high in calorie-dense processed foods and beverages results in abdominal obesity, which, in turn, increases insulin resistance and exaggerates the postprandial spikes in the blood levels of glucose and triglycerides, and, in so doing, also increases systemic inflammation. Abdominal obesity also tends to increase cortisol levels, which causes cravings for calorie-dense foods and predisposes one to further deposition of fat in the abdominal cavity. Thus, the most important dietary change for improving

MetSyn is to reduce daily caloric intake. This will help to eliminate excess intra-abdominal fat, improve all of the other features of MetSyn, and reduce systemic oxidative stress.

POSTPRANDIAL SPIKES IN GLUCOSE AND TRIGLYCERIDES CAUSE OXIDATIVE STRESS AND INFLAMMATION

The high-calorie, high-glycemic diet prevalent in the United States, and increasingly throughout the world, predisposes people to MetSyn and acute and chronic generalized systemic inflammation. A high–glycemic-load meal rich in sugars and starches that are easily digested

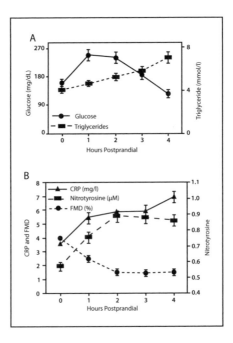

Figure 13.1.

The postprandial rises in glucose and triglycerides trigger immediate proportional rises in free radicals (nitrotyrosine), inflammation (CRP) and lead to deterioration in endothelial function as assessed by flow mediated (FMD).

and quickly absorbed into the bloodstream results in a rapid and steep rise in blood glucose levels. Postprandial hyperglycemia may, in turn, trigger an acute systemic inflammatory response, especially in subjects with metabolic syndrome and/or diabetes (see Chapter 6) (Figure 13.1). When this is repeated regularly, as it is for many American adults and children multiple times each day, it ultimately leads to chronic degenerative diseases and premature aging. Oxidative stress results from high levels of reactive oxygen species (free radicals) that outstrip the body's antioxidant capacities.

These abnormally high blood glucose excursions overwhelm the mitochondrial metabolism, essentially flooding the Krebs cycle with energetic substrate. This exceeds the oxidative phosphorylation buffering capacity, resulting in immediate spikes in the levels of free radicals. These highly reactive oxygen species, such as super-oxide anions, contain oxygen molecules with unpaired electrons. Free radicals are chemically unstable and thus will randomly capture unpaired electrons, thereby binding to chemical moieties in the surrounding biological milieu, resulting in oxidation of compounds in cell membranes, the mitochondria, RNA and DNA, LDL cholesterol, and so on. Oxidation is the same chemical process that rusts iron; it is an important underlying cause of premature aging and contributes to many chronic degenerative diseases.

Although free radicals are a normal byproduct of food metabolism, these pro-oxidants are generated in excess in response to exaggerated spikes in the postprandial blood levels of glucose and fats. This process, called postprandial dysmetabolism, which is present in most individuals with MetSyn and type 2 diabetes, can overwhelm the body's antioxidant capacity. Excess free radical production causes endothelial dysfunction and promotes inflammation throughout the body and, in so doing, predisposes to many common chronic degenerative diseases, including atherosclerosis, diabetes, Alzheimer's disease, cancer, cataracts, macular degeneration, and many types of cancer (Figure 13.2).

DIETARY STRATEGIES TO REDUCE METABOLIC SYNDROME, INFLAMMATION, AND CHRONIC DEGENERATIVE DISEASES

The antioxidant capacity of blood is a measure of its capability to neutralize the potentially damaging pro-oxidant molecules called free radicals. Eating a meal low in antioxidants, such as one high in easily digestible calories and low in refined carbohydrates, animal proteins, and saturated fats, will predictably reduce the blood's antioxidant capacity and induce oxidative stress. Strategies to reduce diet-induced oxidative stress involve blunting the excessive rises in postprandial glucose and triglyceride levels and increasing the intake of dietary antioxidants in the form of plant-based phytonutrients found in vegetables, fruits, nuts, legumes, tea, coffee, wine, and so on. The antioxidants in colorful plant foods and beverages such as berries, greens, carrots, tomatoes, apples, citrus fruits, tea, coffee, and red wine can help reduce meal-generated free radicals and oxidative stress. Additionally, antioxidants found in plant-based foods confer anti-inflammatory benefits by favorably altering genetic transcription factors.

High-glycemic diets, especially in the setting of abdominal obesity and MetSyn, will gener-ate excessive postprandial spikes in blood glucose, which will generate high levels of free radicals,

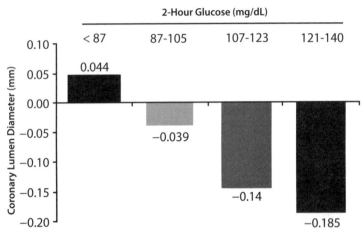

Figure 13.2.

The 2-hour postglucose challenge change in blood glucose was associated with change in coronary artery luminal diameter in a prospective 2-year trial on nondiabetic postmenopausal females. When the postchallenge glucose remained below approximately 100 mg/dL, no progression in coronary stenosis was seen.

which, in turn, promote inflammation, ultimately causing chronic degenerative diseases. This generalized inflammatory response to a high-calorie, high-glycemic diet is exacerbated by excess weight (specifically increased amounts of intra-abdominal fat tissue), a sedentary lifestyle, and conditions characterized by high levels of cortisol and catecholamines, such as emotional and/or physical stress and sleep deprivation.

Steps that will lower postprandial spikes in blood levels of glucose and triglycerides include reducing excess abdominal fat to achieve ideal weight and waist measurements, decreasing serving sizes, and increasing daily physical activity. Additionally, the following specific dietary strategies are highly effective for improving MetSyn, postprandial dysmetabolism, and CV risk factors and prognosis.

LOW-GLYCEMIC DIETS REDUCE OXIDATIVE STRESS AND IMPROVE METABOLIC SYNDROME

A low-glycemic diet will blunt postprandial glucose excursions and result in significantly higher levels of total antioxidant capacity than a high-glycemic diet. A low-glycemic diet will also improve other standard CV risk factors, such as HDL and triglyceride levels. Thus, a diet low in sugars and refined starches (low-carbohydrate diet) will help to reduce the endogenous production of excess levels of free radicals, thereby reducing inflammation, which may lower the incidence of many chronic degenerative diseases.

THE HUNTER-GATHERER DIET

Studies suggest that the hunter-gatherer style of diet may be useful for the prevention and treatment of the MetSyn. One study showed a high prevalence of calcified plaques in the aortas of 3,000-year-old mummies. This fascinating study was widely misinterpreted by the general media as evidence that atherosclerosis is a common and natural age-related human condition. However, a 10-year observational study of 2,500 Greenland Inuit living an indigenous hunter-forager lifestyle during the middle of the last century documented the absence of MIs and other manifestations of cardiovascular disease. The available data suggests that atherosclerosis is a disease of civilization, whereby the abandonment of the hunter-forager lifestyle and the adoption of agriculture is associated with the development of CV disease.

A variety of dietary modifications that were introduced during the Neolithic and Industrial eras may promote chronic low-level vascular inflammation, a well-established mechanism underlying atherosclerosis. The diet of individuals living in agricultural societies, even as long ago as ancient Egypt, was likely based on grains and domesticated animals, which, in contrast to the native hunter-forager diet, had reduced intakes of cardioprotective dietary elements, including omega-3 fatty acids, folic acid, vitamin B6, antioxidants, phytochemicals, and lean proteins. A recent 3-month randomized crossover trial demonstrated that a modern-day "Paleolithic" diet improved multiple indices of MetSyn and cardiovascular risk in type 2 diabetics when compared to a standard "diabetic" diet.

Today's society is characterized by sedentary lifestyles, tobacco use, and the widespread availability of calorie-dense nutritionally depleted foods that magnify the risk of CV disease. However, the nutritional seeds of atherosclerosis had sprouted and were already discernible among ancient Egyptians who had transitioned away from the indigenous diet for which humans were, and remain today, genetically adapted.

The indigenous human diet had much higher levels of omega-3 fatty acids; beneficial plant-based compounds, such as vitamins and antioxidant phytonutrients; fiber; potassium; and lean protein (and hence dietary cholesterol) than our modern diet, but contained much lower levels of sugar, sodium, and saturated fat. Prospective dietary intervention studies have shown a low-carbohydrate Paleolithic-type diet to be effective for weight loss and for improving multiple CV risk factors, including blood pressure, blood glucose, LDL and HDL cholesterol, and triglycerides.

The major drawback of the hunter-gatherer diet relates to the high consumption of animal protein. Although the evidence suggests that most hunter-gatherer cultures consumed 50% or more of their calories from animal sources, these foods were very different from most modern animal-based foods. The land animals, fish, seafood, eggs, insects, and so on were wild and largely unprocessed. The saturated fat content was lower, the omega-3 fatty acid content was higher, and preservatives, such as nitrites and salt, were not used. Even hunter-gatherer cultures, such as the Inuit, who consumed nearly 100% of their calories from wild animal sources, had total cholesterol levels and blood pressures that were very low by modern standards. Indeed, animal proteins and fats tend to be more satiating than easily digestible carbohydrate sources of calories.

Hunter-gatherers consumed the bones of their animal prey whenever possible. Because modern followers of the Paleolithic diet are unlikely to consume bones and are encouraged to avoid dairy products, they might benefit from a daily calcium supplement. Indeed, one intervention trial found that a Paleolithic-type diet induced adverse changes in calcium metabolism.

Thus, animal sources of food are a natural and essential part of the omnivorous human diet. However, a diet high in fatty meat and/or highly processed animal foods tends to be both atherogenic and carcinogenic. The answer to this paradox is to consume modest serving sizes of healthy forms of animal foods, such as egg whites, fish and seafood, skinless chicken breasts, game meats, and lean red meat that is not burned (cooking meat at high temperatures produces carcinogens). It is also very important to consume, in conjunction with the healthy animal foods, a variety of colorful plant produce with each meal.

THE MEDITERRANEAN DIET

The Mediterranean cuisine is not a specific diet but rather a set of eating habits that are traditionally followed by the inhabitants of the Mediterranean region. Sixteen nations surround the Mediterranean Sea, and, although the eating traditions vary widely from one country to the next, these cultures typically follow these general dietary principles:

- High intake of fruits, vegetables, beans, nuts, seeds, and cereal grains

- Use of olive oil for cooking and dressings

- Moderate amounts of fish and seafood but sparse intake of meat

- Low-to-moderate amounts of full-fat cheese and yogurt

- Moderate consumption of wine, typically with meals

- Preference for local, seasonal produce

- Physically active lifestyle usually incorporated into activities of daily life

A 4-year study of a large cohort of people living in Greece reported that following the Mediterranean diet conferred protection against both heart disease and cancer. Overall, those individuals who adhered to the Mediterranean dietary principles most closely were 25% less likely to die during the course of the study.

Investigators from the Framingham Heart Study found that a diet consistent with the fundamentals of the Mediterranean-style diet appears to prevent development of MetSyn. Specifically, a diet high in vegetables, fruit, nuts, omega-3 fatty acids, olive oil, and whole grains but low in refined carbohydrates, saturated fats, and trans fats was associated with avoidance of MetSyn traits, including abdominal obesity, atherogenic dyslipidemia, and insulin resistance. The investigators followed 2,730 participants without diabetes in the Framingham Heart Study Offspring Cohort, mean age 54 years, for an average of 7 years, watching for the development of MetSyn traits. Each participant was evaluated on a Mediterranean-style dietary pattern score, which graded individuals according to consumption of 13 food groups. A higher compliance with the Mediterranean diet principles was associated with significantly lower levels of insulin resistance, waist circumference, fasting glucose, and triglycerides and higher HDL cholesterol levels, after adjusting for potential confounders. Individuals in the highest quartile of Mediterranean diet compliance were 25% less likely to have developed MetSyn than those in the lowest quartile. Thus, the Mediterranean-style diet reduced the likelihood of developing MetSyn during the course of this 7-year prospective observational study.

Studies have evaluated the specific components of the Mediterranean diet to see which ones were most important for conferring the health benefits associated with the consumption of this traditional cuisine. Vogel and colleagues identified the antioxidant-rich foods and beverages, such as vegetables, fruits, olive oil, and red wine, along with foods rich in omega-3s, including fish and nuts, as the important dietary factors for improving CV risk factors and endothelial function.

A more recent epidemiological study of 23,500 Greek adults reported that intake of vegetables, fruits, nuts, legumes, and olive oil and drinking light-to-moderate amounts of alcohol while not consuming a lot of meat or excessive amounts of alcohol was linked to improved longevity. The proportion of the overall improvement in longevity attributable to each of the specific components of the Mediterranean diet were as follows: moderate ethanol consumption, 24%; low consumption of meat and meat products, 17%; high vegetable consumption, 16%; high fruit and nut consumption, 11%; high monounsaturated-to-saturated lipid ratio, 11%; and high legume consumption, 10%.

A controlled dietary trial randomized 215 patients with newly diagnosed type 2 diabetes to either a Mediterranean diet or a low-fat diet. The Mediterranean diet emphasized a high intake of vegetables and whole grains; instead of red meat, participants were advised to eat poultry and fish, with at least 30% of calories derived from fat, principally in the form of olive oil. The low-fat diet, based on American Heart Association (AHA) guidelines, emphasized whole grains and restricted intake of sweets, fats, and high-fat snacks, with a goal of less than 30% of calories from fat. After 4 years, with ongoing dietary counseling, only 44% of newly diagnosed diabetic patients randomized to the Mediterranean diet versus 70% of those randomized to the low-fat AHA diet required glucose-lowering drug therapy for control of their diabetes. Individuals following the Mediterranean diet also showed greater improvement in several cardiovascular risk factors.

Another epidemiological study of over 13,000 people found that those who followed a Mediterranean-style diet were less likely to develop new-onset diabetes. The benefits were especially pronounced in those who were at higher risk of developing type 2 diabetes due to issues such as MetSyn, excess weight, family history, and blood pressure. Study participants with the best adherence to Mediterranean dietary principles had a greater than 50% decrease in the risk of developing diabetes at 4.4 years follow-up.

In summary, following the traditional Mediterranean-style diet results in a lower risk of developing MetSyn, lower blood glucose levels, and a reduced risk of developing type 2 diabetes. The Mediterranean-style diet has also been shown to improve multiple CV risk factors, including abdominal obesity compared to other diets.

IMPORTANCE OF ANTIOXIDANT FOODS IN A MIXED MEAL

Foods rich in antioxidants blunt the levels of free radicals and oxidative stress generated by the consumption of calorie-dense meals high in refined carbohydrates, fats, and proteins. Antioxidant-rich fruits such as blueberries, kiwifruit, grapefruit, and others have been shown to improve the blood antioxidant capacity during the critical early postprandial hours. Importantly, these antioxidant-rich fruits blunt oxidation most effectively when they are eaten as part of a meal, or immediately after a meal, rather than when consumed alone. Thus, eating antioxidant-rich plants during meals reduces the oxidative stress associated with the metabolism of the consumed foods. However, both the timing and the types of food consumed are important to minimize oxidative stress. The antioxidants abundant in deeply hued plant foods help to blunt the oxidative stress inherent in the metabolism of calories, but these free radical scavengers are relatively transient in the bloodstream; thus, they should be eaten as part of a mixed meal.

Phytochemicals in foods and beverages have variable bioavailability and antioxidant capacity and are typically cleared from the blood within 2 to 4 hours of consumption. Thus, an individual should ideally consume antioxidant-rich foods and/or beverages with each meal and snack to ensure that the body has a steady supply of blood-borne antioxidants to help buffer and eliminate postprandial oxidative stress throughout the day. In general, the requirement for dietary antioxidants is directly proportional to the number of calories consumed. Typically, about two and a half servings of antioxidant-containing vegetables and/or fruits during a meal will markedly diminish oxidative stress following the meal.

Furthermore, studies show that certain foods help to slow the digestion and absorption after a meal. For instance, the addition of lean protein, high-fiber foods, nuts (especially tree nuts such as walnuts, almonds, and pecans), vinegar, or one or two (but not more) alcoholic drinks has been shown to significantly reduce the postprandial spike in glucose, which is directly correlated with the rise in free radicals and oxidative–stress-induced inflammation. When fruit is consumed with a meal containing protein and/or nuts, the antioxidants present in the fruit and nuts will help to reduce oxidative stress, and the protein will help to slow absorption of the calories, which will blunt the postprandial spikes in glucose and triglycerides.

Fish, more specifically the omega-3 fatty acids present in fish oil, have been shown to reduce postprandial triglycerides, which appear to be an important CV risk factor (more so than fasting triglyceride levels). Marine sources of omega-3 fatty acids will also reduce systemic inflammation, possibly in part by their beneficial effects on postmeal triglyceride levels.

COFFEE, CINNAMON, DAIRY PRODUCTS AND METABOLIC SYNDROME

An inverse relationship between coffee intake and the development of type 2 diabetes was observed in the Nurses' Health Study, a Dutch population study, and a Japanese study, where the consumption of coffee was also inversely associated with the manifestations of MetSyn. In Holland, drinking at least three cups of coffee or tea per day was shown to be associated with a lower risk of type 2 diabetes, and this lower risk could not be explained by potassium or caffeine intake or changes in blood pressure. In a U.S. study, decreased development of type 2 diabetes was shown to be related to the number of cups of coffee that were consumed each day, irrespective of whether the coffee was decaffeinated, filtered, or instant.

The effects of coffee on insulin sensitivity are thought to be mediated through an increased expression of mitochondrial uncoupling proteins. Therefore, independent of the effect of caffeine, coffee consumption appears to decrease the risk of developing MetSyn and diabetes by improving insulin resistance.

One study found that cinnamon ingestion over a 2-week period in normal volunteers not only improved glucose tolerance, but also lowered insulin levels and insulin resistance. Cinnamon lowers postprandial glucose better than fasting glucose. Cinnamon has also been shown in subjects with MetSyn to improve systolic blood pressure and decrease total body fat. The chromium and polyphenols in cinnamon are thought to lead to improvements in the manifestations of MetSyn.

Regular use of dairy products also improves the manifestations of MetSyn. In over 40,000 males in the Health Professionals Follow-Up Study, over a 12-year period, when adjusted for confounders, those in the top quintile for dairy product intake had a 23% significant reduction in the development of type 2 diabetes compared with the bottom quintile. However, if high-fat milk was used, there was no reduction in the risk of developing diabetes, but for each daily serving of low-fat milk there was a 12% reduction. Although there was no interaction in this study with the BMI, a high dairy intake not only decreased blood pressure, but also decreased the risk of stroke and other CV events. In addition, with a high dairy intake the rate of development of colon cancer was decreased, but for unknown reasons there was an increase in the incidence of prostate cancer. Because both of these cancers are associated with MetSyn (see Chapter 11), this discrepancy is surprising. Therefore, utilizing low-fat dairy products results in improvements in the manifestations of MetSyn and a decreased risk of diabetes, cardiac events, and colon cancer.

ALCOHOL AND METABOLIC SYNDROME

Alcohol is an underrecognized insulin sensitizer. One glass of red wine immediately before or with the evening meal will reduce postprandial glucose by approximately 30% in healthy adults, as well as in those with MetSyn and type 2 diabetes (Figure 13.3). One drink of other types of alcohol will lower the postprandial glucose about 20%. This is a transient effect, which is why a daily habit of light-to-moderate alcohol intake with the evening meal is the

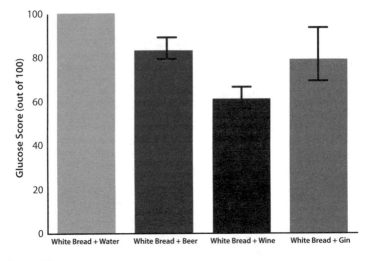

Figure 13.3.

Light to moderate alcohol consumption with the evening meal significantly reduces post prandial glucose. This effect was more prominent with red wine compared with gin or beer.

drinking pattern that is most strongly correlated with improved long-term health measures. Because the magnitude of postprandial glucose excursion is directly correlated with free radical production and systemic inflammation, daily light-to-moderate drinking lowers chronic risks not only for CAD, but also for MetSyn, type 2 diabetes, stroke, dementia, and HF. Physicians who drink one to two drinks per day decrease their chances of developing diabetes by 43%. In other studies, one or two alcoholic drinks will reduce the likelihood of developing type 2 diabetes by about 30% compared to nondrinkers. Other manifestations of MetSyn, such as a low HDL level, an increased PAI_1 level, and enhanced platelet aggregation, are also improved with light-to-moderate intake. In multiple epidemiological studies, alcohol, probably, in part, through its effects on the manifestations of MetSyn, decreases cardiac events by 30%, and both cardiac and all-cause mortality rates by approximately 20%.

In the Wisconsin Retinopathy Study, type 2 diabetic subjects who averaged more than one drink per day decreased their mortality by 89% compared with type 2 diabetic subjects who had never utilized alcohol. In the Nurses' Health Study of over 5,000 diabetic subjects, of whom 295 had had a cardiac event, those diabetic nurses who averaged over a half of an alcoholic drink per day were 52% less likely to have had a cardiac event. Similarly, in the Physician's Health Study, the mortality among diabetic physicians who utilized alcohol on a daily basis was 58% less than in those physicians who had never used alcohol. Therefore, one to two drinks per day in the diabetic male and a one-half a drink per day in the diabetic female will not only improve the manifestations of MetSyn but also reduce CV risks as well as CV events and mortality. In women, if alcohol is limited to a half drink per day the risk of breast cancer is not increased.

If the alcoholic beverage is taken with the evening meal, the risk of alcohol-induced hypoglycemia, which is caused by alcohol acutely decreasing hepatic gluconeogenesis and hepatic glucose production, is nullified. However, the effect of alcohol on decreasing gluconeogenesis and hepatic glucose production also reduces postprandial hyperglycemia. The rise in glucose following a meal in the diabetic patient is often due to the continued release of glucagon on hepatic glucose release, which should be suppressed with eating but is not because of decreased effect of GLP_1, which is released by the K cells of the ileum. Light-to-moderate alcohol consumption also improves insulin sensitivity and glucose uptake by the skeletal muscles for 12 to 24 hours, which also contribute to ethanol's favorable effects on postmeal glucose levels. Lowering of postprandial glucose has been shown to be associated with decreased atherogenesis and decreased cardiac events and is an unrecognized and important component of alcohol's cardioprotective effect.

One alcoholic drink is defined as 12 ounces of beer, 5 ounces of wine, or 1.5 ounces of liquor or distilled spirits. For most health measures, red wine appears to confer the strongest benefits. At intakes of one-half to two drinks per day, the type of alcohol that is utilized is less important, although with higher intakes wine might be safer than liquor/spirits or beer. The incidence of many adverse health effects, including cancer, stroke, hypertension, heart failure, arrhythmias, and dementia, increase proportionally at intakes over two drinks per day.

ARTIFICIAL SWEETENERS

The TIR2/RIR3 taste receptor detects sucrose at concentrations above 1 part per 200, whereas bitter substances are detected if present in only a few parts per million. Therefore, most humans prefer "sweet" rather than "bitter" foods. If the "sweet food" is a fruit, this preference for sweet foods does not lead to obesity and/or the MetSyn. For example, a 8-ounce apple, as well as continuing more vitamins and minerals, contains fewer calories than 2 ounces of bread. Furthermore, fruits induce satiety more readily than bread because of their low energy density, low glycemic index, and high fiber content.

However, when sucrose and high-fructose corn syrup are refined, concentrated, and consumed in large amounts, serum glucose and insulin levels are elevated due to increased insulin resistance. As a result, triglycerides, inflammatory mediators, and reactive oxygen radicals are elevated. Therefore, an increased intake of refined carbohydrates increases the risk of developing diabetes and cardiovascular disease because it is lacking in fiber and antioxidants.

An overrated solution to excess consumption of refined carbohydrate is the use of artificial sweeteners, such as saccharin, acesulfame, aspartamate, neotame, sucralose, or stevia. However, these "sweeteners" result in much more intense (hundreds- to thousands-fold) sensation of sweetness. Of particular concern is the use of sweeteners in drinks that contain no calories, unlike other artificially sweetened foods that contain other nutrients. Diet drinks are typically consumed without food, the result being a dissociation between sweet taste and calorie intake. This dissociation has the potential to disrupt the hormonal and neurobehavioral pathways that regulate the feelings of hunger and satiety. For example, rodents that were fed saccharin when compared with those that were fed glucose increased calorie intake and increased body weight. Furthermore, rodents faced with the choice of intravenous cocaine or oral saccharin preferred oral saccharin, even if the animals had previously been exposed to cocaine. Thus, the desire for sweetness through chronic use of artificial sweeteners may be an addiction greater than that caused by exposure to cocaine or other addictive drugs.

No prospective studies of diet drink consumption, body weight, and MetSyn have been conducted in humans. However, in the San Antonio Heart Study in 5,158 adults over 7 years the consumption of diet drinks was proportional to increases in measurements of obesity. In the Multi-Ethnic Study of Atherosclerosis (MESA), the consumption of more than 21 diet drinks per week resulted in a twofold increased risk of developing obesity when compared with those subjects who did not consume diet drinks. Furthermore, in this study daily consumption of diet drinks resulted in a 36% increased risk of developing the MetSyn and a 62% increased risk of developing type 2 diabetes. However, reverse causation may be a factor in this study, because weight gain may result in increased utilization of diet drinks.

How can diet drinks, which are utilized to decrease body weight, result in weight gain? Over time, calories displaced by artificial sweetness may be replaced from other sources. In addition, overstimulation of taste (TIR2/RIR3) receptors by frequent utilization of intense sweeteners may result in a reversion to an infantile state, where tolerances to other, more complex tastes are lost. Furthermore, less intensely sweet but more satisfying foods such as fruits and vegetables may become less palatable, and the quality of the diet may shift to foods that induce weight gain and the MetSyn.

Artificial sweeteners have been used for over a century and have been shown not to increase the risk of cancer. Recently, publicity regarding the effects of refined sugar and marketing by manufacturers of products containing artificial sweeteners has led to an increased intake of artificial sweeteners, especially in the form of diet drinks. The intake of diet drinks has increased from 1 ounce per day per person in 1960 to 4 ounces per day per person in the first decade of the twenty-first century. However, in those who regularly use diet drinks the consumption is in excess of 24 oz per day.

Although in recent years multiple synthetic additives have been utilized in the manufacture of foods, artificial sweeteners, especially when utilized in beverages, have developed a prominence because of their affinity to interact with ancient sensioneural pathways. This effect, rather than the desired result of decreasing body weight, might paradoxically result in weight gain, increased insulin resistance, and worsening of the MetSyn.

DRUGS THAT IMPROVE METABOLIC SYNDROME

Use of RAAS blockers improve the manifestations of MetSyn. In the HOPE study, the ACE inhibitor ramipril decreased the incidence of developing diabetes by 30%, and in the SOLVD study the ACE inhibitor enalapril decreased the development of diabetes by 74%.

As far as ARBs are concerned, trandolapril reduced the development of diabetes in the PEACE study by 17%; candesartan in the SCOPE and CHARM studies decreased the development of diabetes by 19% and 22%, respectively. In the LIFE trial, losartan, compared to atenolol, reduced the risk of diabetes by 25%.

Aldosterone blockers such as eplerenone and spironoloactone, at least in animal studies, improve insulin resistance, probably because high aldosterone levels have been shown to suppress insulin signaling by downregulating insulin receptor substrate 1 (IRS_1). The new direct renin inhibitor, aliskiren, has also been shown to lower insulin resistance and oxidative stress.

By their vasodilatory action, alpha blockers reduce insulin resistance, and when used in combination with a beta blocker are termed "vasodilating beta blockers." Vasoconstricting beta blockers decrease the surface area for absorption of glucose and increase insulin resistance, whereas vasodilating blockers increase the surface area for glucose absorption and lower insulin resistance by as much as 20%.

In the West of Scotland study, pravastatin decreased the risk of developing diabetes by 30%. However, studies with other statins have not shown a similar effect, and a meta-analysis of statin studies showed that, with the exception of pravastatin, statins increase insulin resistance. In fact, in the JUPITER study rosuvastatin increased the rate of new-onset diabetes.

Xanthine oxidoreductase inhibition by drugs such as allopurinol, which is used in the treatment of gout, reduce insulin resistance and the manifestations of MetSyn. In a study of subjects with MetSyn, allopurinol reduced oxidative stress and improved endothelial function without significantly decreasing CRP and fibrinogen levels. In an animal study in which the manifestations of MetSyn were induced with a high-fructose diet, allopurinol and captopril monotherapy both reduced the features of MetSyn. A combination of these two drugs synergistically reduced the features of MetSyn, including hypertension, insulin resistance, and dyslipidemia. It has been postulated that an elevated uric acid level, through its effect on endothelial function, may precipitate or even worsen the manifestations of MetSyn. The new nonpurine and selective xanthine oxidase inhibitor febuxostat has been shown to not only significantly lower uric acid levels, but also to significantly lower blood pressure, triglycerides, and insulin levels in a randomized animal study of fructose-induced MetSyn.

It has always been recognized that a high uric acid level was at least a marker for both MetSyn and an increased risk of MI. High insulin levels have been shown to suppress uric acid excretion, and hyperuricemia is independently associated with higher insulin levels. Although hyperuricemia is also associated with elevated FFAs and triglycerides, correction of this hyperlipidemia has no effect on uric acid levels. Thus, an increased uric acid level may occur as a result of hyperinsulinemia and MetSyn but can cause or worsen MetSyn.

CONCLUSIONS

Elimination of excess calorie intake is the single most important dietary factor for preventing or treating MetSyn. It will help to reduce intra-abdominal adipose tissue—the most important manifestation and cause of MetSyn. Additionally, avoidance of high-glycemic foods and beverages and other easily digestible, highly processed, calorie-dense foods and beverages is important. The consumption of foods and beverages with added sugar, high-fructose corn syrup, and artificial sweeteners should be minimized. Ideally, a modest serving size of lean fresh animal protein should be eaten at two meals daily and vegetable protein such as nuts or legumes should be consumed at least once daily. Two or three servings of vegetables and fruits (ideally those high in antioxidants and low in calories) should be eaten at each of the three daily meals. One alcoholic drink (red wine with or before the evening meal is ideal) will blunt postprandial glucose excursion and reduce risk of MetSyn, type 2 diabetes, and CV diseases. Other specific foods and beverages that may be useful in preventing or treating MetSyn include coffee, nonfat or low-fat dairy, cinnamon, vinegar, fish and fish oil, whole grains and other high-fiber foods, and olive oil.

Weight loss, exercise, light-to-moderate alcohol consumption, as well as increased intake of dairy products, coffee, and cinnamon have been shown to have a positive effect on the manifestations of MetSyn. RAAS, vasodilating alpha, and beta blockers may also lead to improvements in insulin resistance and MetSyn.

Chapter 14

Metabolic Syndrome: Yesterday, Today, and Tomorrow

MetSyn developed to protect the "hunter-gatherer" from starvation. Those who inherited the genes for MetSyn (thrifty phenotype) survived by storing energy in the form of fat so that during periods of famine sufficient energy to survive was available. Thus, primitive man, through developing MetSyn, was better adapted to withstand periods of starvation and drought, as were his offspring.

Moving forward to the twenty-first century, there is no shortage of calories, at least in industrialized societies. Furthermore, opportunities for exercise have decreased significantly. This decrease in exercise combined with a plentiful supply of inexpensive food with a high saturated fat and fructose content has resulted in an epidemic of obesity. The inherited trend to develop MetSyn has been activated by changes in lifestyle and obesity, which has led to epidemics of cardiac disease and type 2 diabetes. Furthermore, as life expectancy increases, aging of the population further exacerbates not only MetSyn, but also the incidence and prevalence of type 2 diabetes and cardiac disease. Thus, MetSyn, which originally provided survival advantages to our Paleolithic hunter-gatherer ancestors, has now become a health liability in the modern high-calorie, sedentary milieu.

Initially, MetSyn was recognized as being associated with type 2 diabetes and later with heart disease. However, we now recognize that the manifestations of MetSyn are protean, adversely affecting the quality and quantity of life in many ways. The risks of cancer and AD are increased with MetSyn. Hepatic adenocarcinoma and hepatic failure occur more frequently with MetSyn because of its association with the nonalcoholic fatty liver diseases. In women, infertility, pregnancy-induced hypertension, preeclamptic toxemia, and androgenation all add to the morbidity caused by MetSyn. Increased morbidity also occurs in the male, where MetSyn is associated with testosterone deficiency and BPH. Kidney stones, renal decompensation, peripheral neuropathy, sleep apnea, decreased exercise tolerance, all of which are associated with MetSyn, worsen quality of life and increase mortality.

What of the future? It is now estimated that children born in the twenty-first century into cultures with healthy diets/lifestyles, such as the Mediterranean French and the Okinawans, will have a 50% chance of living to a hundred years of age. It is also estimated that a third of those individuals born into the current millennium will develop diabetes before they die. Indeed, if the babies are members of minority groups that have an increased prevalence of diabetes, half of them are predicted to develop diabetes in their lifetime.

Furthermore, because of continuing lifestyle changes, diabetes is occurring at a younger and younger age, especially in the obese and in minority groups. Nowadays, 10% of children who develop diabetes before age 20 have type 2 rather than type 1 diabetes. In high-risk minority groups, diabetes developing before the age of 20 is type 2 in 50% of cases.

Developing diabetes at a younger age and living longer due to other health improvements means that the chances of developing diabetic complications is greatly increased, and it is the cost of diabetic complications that accounts for the enormous national and international expenditure on diabetes.

The advances that have been made in preventing cardiac events by decreasing blood pressure, treating hyperlipidemia, utilizing antiplatelet therapies, and decreasing the frequency of cigarette smoking may well be neutralized by the escalating prevalence of MetSyn with its associated CV risk factors.

So, what can we do? We can certainly treat the components of MetSyn and, in diabetic patients, MetSyn itself. By treating MetSyn in the prediabetic individual, we may even be able to decrease not only the risk of developing diabetes but also the incidence of CV events and cancer. However, we must educate our patients that the best strategy to prevent obesity, diabetes, and CV events is to initiate changes in diet and lifestyle, preferably at a young age.

Unfortunately, in the long term we cannot get most patients to lose weight and maintain a healthy weight chronically. We also do not have drugs that meaningfully help decrease calorie intake or in other ways treat obesity. Likewise, many patients enthusiastically start an exercise program only to become distracted and unmotivated before they develop the habit of a daily fitness regimen. Should we be resorting to gastric bypass surgery to obtain our goals? Very significant weight loss can be achieved and sustained with gastric lap banding and other bariatric surgical procedures, and gastric bypass surgery is associated with prompt resolution of type 2 diabetes in 70% of patients. However the cost of treating every patient with a BMI of over 40 or a diabetic patient with a BMI of over 35 with bariatric surgery would be prohibitive.

The epidemics of obesity, MetSyn, type 2 diabetes, CV disease, and cancer are, in part, manifestations of maladaptive lifestyles and diets inherent in the modern civilized world that are at odds with our genetic identity. Although the human race has dealt with epidemics of acute infectious diseases, we have not previously faced an epidemic of chronic disease on a scale the likes of which we are currently experiencing. This is particularly relevant because the cost of treating an epidemic of a chronic disease is much higher. In fact, the cost of treating the epidemic of obesity, MetSyn, type 2 diabetes, CV disease, and cancer may well be unsustainable for many countries and could potentially overwhelm available resources and paralyze health-care systems.

As physicians dealing with individual patients we must enthusiastically endorse dietary and exercise measures to prevent or reverse obesity and insulin resistance. We must also serve as role models through exhibiting these healthy lifestyle and dietary behaviors. Additionally, we must help coordinate national and international efforts by governments and the World Health Organization to educate the population on the need to prevent these chronic diseases and at the same time provide incentives for the individuals to exercise and obtain and maintain ideal body weight. Otherwise, we will have to deal with the potentially devastating consequences at both the personal and societal levels.